The Beginner's Guide to Intensive Care

A Handbook for Junior Doctors and Allied Professionals

The Beginner's Guide to Intensive Care

A Handbook for Junior Doctors and Allied Professionals
Second Edition

Edited by
Nitin Arora
Shondipon K. Laha

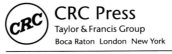

CRC Press
Taylor & Francis Group
Boca Raton London New York

CRC Press is an imprint of the
Taylor & Francis Group, an **informa** business

CRC Press
Taylor & Francis Group
6000 Broken Sound Parkway NW, Suite 300
Boca Raton, FL 33487-2742

© 2018 by Taylor & Francis Group, LLC
CRC Press is an imprint of Taylor & Francis Group, an Informa business

No claim to original U.S. Government works

Printed on acid-free paper

International Standard Book Number-13: 978-0-8153-8321-5 (Hardback)
International Standard Book Number-13: 978-1-138-03578-2 (Paperback)

Visit the Taylor & Francis Web site at
http://www.taylorandfrancis.com

and the CRC Press Web site at
http://www.crcpress.com

CV 07.14.2020 1218

Contents

Foreword

In this introduction to intensive care medicine (ICM), Arora and Laha have provided a very useful overview of what it means to be an intensive care clinician, whether physician, nurse, or allied health professional. We are the acute general practitioners of hospital medicine. We care for patients with life-threatening acute illnesses, for patients with severe chronic disease, and for their families at what is often the most difficult time of their lives. To do this we have to work collaboratively, across disciplines, at pace, often multitasking, synthesising large volumes of data into information, and transforming information into action. This demands high-level technical and non-technical skills. For the beginner, it is usually the technical elements which are the most obvious challenge at first, but with acquisition of expertise these become part of the background, and it is the non-technical skills which come to the fore – learning to listen, to work as a team, to minimise error, to relieve suffering.

These elements are all components of the competency-based training programme in ICM (https://ficm.ac.uk/training-examinations/curriculum-assessment-training), which was approved by the General Medical Council in 2011 thereby making ICM a primary speciality. The review board was impressed by the multidisciplinary nature of the programme, the firm emphasis on research and evidence-based practice, and co-design with patients and relatives through CoBaTrICE (http://www.cobatrice.org/en/index.asp). These features are reflected in this book, which provides an excellent introduction to the management of acute illness for all clinical staff, and a solid foundation for those who choose to make ICM a fulfilling lifelong career.

Julian Bion, FRCP, FRCA, FFICM, MD
Professor of Intensive Care Medicine
University of Birmingham
Founding Dean
Faculty of Intensive Care Medicine

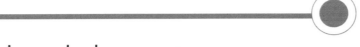

Acknowledgements

We would like to thank all the medical and nursing staff working in critical care at University Hospitals Birmingham NHS Foundation Trust, and Lancashire Teaching Hospitals NHS Foundation Trust. Thanks to my wife Ira for her support, encouragement and patience over the years.

Nitin

I would like to thank my wife Alex and my parents with their unswerving support over many decades. I hope my kids, Jonny, Ned and Meg benefit from the ever rapidly developing technology that means the medicine in this book will be out of date by the time they come of age.

Shond

Editors

Dr Nitin Arora, FRCA, FRCPE, DICM, FFICM, is a Consultant in Intensive Care Medicine and Anaesthesia at University Hospitals Birmingham NHS Foundation Trust, Birmingham. He has previously worked in medicine, intensive care and anaesthesia in India and the United Kingdom.

Dr Shondipon K. Laha, BM, BCh, MA, FRCA, FFICM, is a Consultant in Intensive Care Medicine and Anaesthesia at Lancashire Teaching Hospitals NHS Foundation Trust. He read medicine at Oxford University and completed dual specialty training in anaesthesia and intensive care medicine in the North West of England.

Contributors

Aoife Abbey
Specialty Registrar Intensive
    Care Medicine
West Midlands

Nafeesa Akhtar
Specialty Registrar Anaesthesia
West Midlands

Fayaz Baba
Specialty Registrar Anaesthesia
West Midlands

Asfa Bashir
Highly Specialist Speech and
    Language Therapist
University Hospitals Birmingham
    NHS Foundation Trust
Birmingham

Richard Benson
Specialty Registrar Intensive Care
    Medicine and Anaesthesia
North West Deanery

Peter Bunting
Consultant Intensive Care
    Medicine and Anaesthesia
Lancashire Teaching Hospitals
    NHS Foundation Trust
Preston

Sarah Bunting
Intensive Care Medicine
    Physiotherapist
Lancashire Teaching Hospitals
    NHS Foundation Trust
Preston

Shashikumar Chandrashekaraiah
Consultant Intensive Care
    Medicine and Anaesthesia
Lancashire Teaching Hospitals
    NHS Foundation Trust
Preston

Irfan Chaudry
Consultant Intensive Care
    Medicine and Anaesthesia
Lancashire Teaching Hospitals
    NHS Foundation Trust
Preston

Neil Crooks
Consultant Intensive Care
    Medicine and Anaesthesia
University Hospitals Birmingham
    NHS Foundation Trust
Birmingham

Ron Daniels
Consultant Intensive Care
    Medicine and Anaesthesia
University Hospitals Birmingham
    NHS Foundation Trust
Chief Executive UK Sepsis Trust
Birmingham

Angela Day
Specialty Doctor Anaesthesia
University Hospitals Birmingham
    NHS Foundation Trust
Birmingham

Edward Denison-Davies
Consultant Intensive Care
    Medicine and
    Anaesthesia
Lancashire Teaching Hospitals
    NHS Foundation Trust
Preston

Anna Dennis
Consultant Intensive Care
    Medicine and Anaesthesia
University Hospitals Birmingham
    NHS Foundation Trust
Birmingham

Gavin Denton
Advanced Critical Care
    Practitioner
University Hospitals Birmingham
    NHS Foundation Trust
Birmingham

Mike Dickinson
Human Patient Simulator
    Training Coordinator
Lancashire Teaching Hospitals
    NHS Foundation Trust
Preston

Jonathan Downham
Advanced Critical Care Practitioner
South Warwickshire NHS
    Foundation Trust
Warwick

Laura Dyal
Specialty Registrar Anaesthesia
West Midlands

Hozefa Ebrahim
Consultant Intensive Care
    Medicine and Anaesthesia
University Hospitals Birmingham
    NHS Foundation Trust
Birmingham

Michael Elliot
Consultant Intensive Care
    Medicine and Anaesthesia
University Hospitals Birmingham
    NHS Foundation Trust
Birmingham

Robert Fallon
Senior Clinical Fellow
Intensive Care Medicine and
    Anaesthesia
Lancashire Teaching Hospitals
    NHS Foundation Trust
Preston

Helga Fichter
Consultant Intensive Care
    Medicine and Anaesthesia
University Hospitals Birmingham
    NHS Foundation Trust
Birmingham

Emma Foster
Clinical Fellow
University Hospitals Birmingham
    NHS Foundation Trust
Birmingham

Peter Frank
Consultant Intensive Care
    Medicine and
    Anaesthesia
Lancashire Teaching Hospitals
    NHS Foundation Trust
Preston

Catriona Frankling
Specialty Registrar Anaesthesia
West Midlands

Fang Gao
Professor of Anaesthesia
Critical Care and Pain
University of Birmingham
Honorary Consultant Intensive
    Care Medicine
University Hospitals Birmingham
    NHS Foundation Trust
Birmingham

Andrew Gosling
Consultant Anaesthetics and
    Critical Care
Lancashire Teaching Hospitals
    NHS Foundation Trust
Preston

Carl Groves
Core Trainee ACCS
Anaesthesia
West Midlands

Jennifer Hares
Specialty Registrar
    Anaesthesia
West Midlands

Mohammed Hatab
Specialty Registrar Intensive
    Care Medicine and
    Anaesthesia
North West Deanery

Andrew Haughton
Consultant Intensive Care
    Medicine and Anaesthesia
Lancashire Teaching Hospitals
    NHS Foundation Trust
Preston

Anna Herbert
Core Trainee Medicine
North West Deanery

Joseph Herold
Core Trainee Anaesthesia
North West Deanery

Rachel Howarth
Core Trainee Anaesthesia
North West Deanery

Julian Hull
Consultant Intensive Care
    Medicine and Anaesthesia
University Hospitals Birmingham
    NHS Foundation Trust
Birmingham

Arumugam Jagadeeswaran
Consultant Intensive Care
    Medicine and Anaesthesia
University Hospitals Birmingham
    NHS Foundation Trust
Birmingham

Gareth P. Jones
Foundation Doctor
Lancashire Teaching Hospitals
    NHS Foundation Trust
Preston

Paul Johnston
Consultant Intensive Care
    Medicine and Anaesthesia
University Hospitals Birmingham
    NHS Foundation Trust
Birmingham

Sudhindra Kulkarni
Specialty Registrar Intensive Care
    Medicine and Anaesthesia
North West Deanery

Lucie Linhartova
Consultant Intensive Care
    Medicine and Anaesthesia
University Hospitals Birmingham
    NHS Foundation Trust
Birmingham

Kunal Lund
Specialty Registrar Intensive
    Care Medicine and
    Anaesthesia
North West Deanery

Brendan McGrath
Consultant Intensive Care
    Medicine and Anaesthesia
University Hospitals of South
    Manchester
National Tracheostomy Lead
    Clinician
Manchester

Karen Meacher
Specialty Registrar Anaesthesia
West Midlands

Sarah Milton-White
Specialty Registrar Intensive
    Care Medicine and
    Anaesthesia
West Midlands

Robert O'Brien
Consultant Intensive Care
    Medicine and Anaesthesia
University Hospitals Birmingham
    NHS Foundation Trust
Birmingham

Olusegun Olusanya
Clinical Fellow
Intensive Care Medicine
North Hampshire Hospital
Basingstoke

Thomas Owen
Consultant Intensive Care
    Medicine and Anaesthesia
Lancashire Teaching Hospitals
    NHS Foundation Trust
Preston

Adeyemi Oyedele
Critical Care Pharmacist
University Hospitals of Coventry
    and Warwickshire
Coventry

Jonathan Paige
Specialty Registrar Intensive
    Care Medicine and
    Anaesthesia
West Midlands

Nicola Pargeter
Highly Specialist Speech and
    Language Therapist
University Hospitals Birmingham
    NHS Foundation Trust
Birmingham

Daniel Park
Consultant Intensive Care
    Medicine and Anaesthesia
University Hospitals Birmingham
    NHS Foundation Trust
Birmingham

Vanisha Patel
Research Fellow Anaesthesia
University Hospitals Birmingham
    NHS Foundation Trust
Birmingham

Bryony Patrick
Senior Clinical Fellow
Intensive Care Medicine and
    Anaesthesia
Lancashire Teaching Hospitals
    NHS Foundation Trust
Preston

Gavin Perkins
Professor of Critical Care
    Warwick University
Honorary Consultant Intensive
    Care Medicine
University Hospitals Birmingham
    NHS Foundation Trust
Birmingham

Nagendra Pinnampeni
Specialty Registrar Anaesthesia
East Midlands

Nicholas R. Plummer
Core Trainee ACCS
North West Deanery

Mark Pugh
Consultant Intensive Care
    Medicine and Anaesthesia
Lancashire Teaching Hospitals
    NHS Foundation Trust
Preston

Govindan Raghuraman
Consultant Intensive Care
    Medicine and
    Anaesthesia
University Hospitals Birmingham
    NHS Foundation Trust
Birmingham

Eldilla Rizal
Specialty Registrar Paediatric
    Intensive Care Medicine
West Midlands

Naresh Sandur
Consultant Anaesthesia
University Hospitals Birmingham
    NHS Foundation Trust
Birmingham

Amanda Shaw
Consultant Intensive Care
    Medicine and Anaesthesia
Lancashire Teaching Hospitals
    NHS Foundation Trust
Preston

Daniel Shuttleworth
Specialty Registrar Intensive
    Care Medicine and
    Anaesthesia
West Midlands

Ben Slater
Consultant Intensive Care
    Medicine and Anaesthesia
Victoria Hospitals
Kirkcaldy

Craig Spencer
Consultant Intensive Care
    Medicine and Anaesthesia
Lancashire Teaching Hospitals
    NHS Foundation Trust
Preston

James Turner
Research Fellow Anaesthesia
University Hospitals Birmingham
    NHS Foundation Trust
Birmingham

Katherine Turner
Foundation Doctor
Lancashire Teaching Hospitals
    NHS Foundation Trust
Preston

Huw Twamley
Consultant Intensive Care
    Medicine and Anaesthesia
Lancashire Teaching Hospitals
    NHS Foundation Trust
Preston

Ian Tyrell-Marsh
Specialty Registrar Intensive
    Care Medicine and
    Anaesthesia
North West Deanery

Rochelle Velho
Academic Clinical Fellow in
    Critical Care Medicine
CT2 Anaesthesia
West Midlands

Vijay Venkatesh
Specialty Registrar Anaesthesia
West Midlands

Adrian Wong
Consultant Intensive Care
    Medicine and Anaesthesia
Oxford University Hospitals NHS
    Foundation Trust
Oxford

Lucy Wood
Highly Specialist Speech and
    Language Therapist
University Hospitals Birmingham
    NHS Foundation Trust
Birmingham

Ben Wooldridge
Specialty Registrar Anaesthesia
West Midlands

Richard Yardley
Core Trainee ACCS
North West Deanery

Joyce Yeung
Associate Professor in Critical
    Care and Anaesthesia
Warwick University
Honorary Consultant Intensive
    Care Medicine
University Hospitals Birmingham
    NHS Foundation Trust
Birmingham

Introduction

The first edition of this book was published in 2010. As it was a book that was designed to be basic and introductory, we hoped that we would never have to revisit it. However, as time went on, we have been inundated with requests. These were initially minor but it became clear that we needed to give the book an overhaul to keep it relevant.

In the last seven years, we have seen a number of new therapies in intensive care, as well as the rising popularity of imaging modalities like point of care ultrasound.

Intensive care medicine (ICM) has become a stand-alone specialty in the United Kingdom, and we are beginning to understand the psychological burden of intensive care, not just on survivors and families but also on healthcare professionals.

The new edition has been almost completely re-written and greatly expanded. There are new chapters on ultrasound, social media, stress and burnout, research, the ICU team and many others. All chapters have been written by established intensive care consultants or experts in their respective fields. Some skills are best learned at the bedside, so we have limited the length for some chapters while others have more detail.

The previous edition proved to be surprisingly popular with non-medical professionals, and so whilst we have attempted to follow the ICM curriculum for stage-1 training we want this book to also be accessible to the foundation doctor, advanced critical care practitioner or critical care nurse.

This book is not a replacement for the traditional textbooks, but adopts a pragmatic approach to common problems on the unit for both doctors and allied healthcare professionals.

Nitin Arora
Shondipon K. Laha

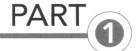

PART 1

BASICS

1

Your first day and what to expect

JAMES TURNER AND JOYCE YEUNG

The idea of your first day working in intensive care can be a daunting prospect. In the remainder of the hospital, the intensive care unit (ICU) is often perceived as a vastly complex world of 'life support', ventilators and inotropes. In reality, with the benefit of time, you will realise that the ICU continues the basic tenets of treatment carried out in the rest of the hospital, except with closer monitoring and some additional interventions, which require a high staff-to-patient ratio. Often, basic medical treatment is continued but with the addition of organ support, to maintain physiology in as normal a state as possible, allowing time for the actual treatment of the underlying condition to work. Using sepsis as an example, the treatment is antimicrobial medication. However, the profound vasodilation and resulting hypotension could result in death before the antibiotics can work. Vasoactive agents are employed to maintain end-organ perfusion while the antibiotics and the patient's own immune system work to combat the cause of the sepsis.

Patients are admitted to the ICU for a number of reasons. Common indications for ICU admission include hypotension unresponsive to fluid resuscitation (e.g. sepsis), myocardial infarction, cardiac arrest, requirement for advanced respiratory support (e.g. severe asthma, COPD exacerbation), requirement for sedation, head injury, status epilepticus, cardiac arrest, severe liver disease, advanced post-operative monitoring due to comorbidities or severity of surgery (e.g. laparotomy, aortic aneurysm repair) and requirement for renal support. This admission may be planned or emergent, with emergencies making up over 75% of admissions. Survival to discharge from critical care varies dramatically depending on the reason for admission and any physiological impairment but is approximately 85%, including elective admissions. Patients admitted from the emergency department have a 71% survival to critical care discharge.

THE 'USUAL' DAY

The first day on the ICU will almost certainly start differently compared to how you have worked in other specialties. The handover from the night team to the day team is a vital part of patient care, and is taken seriously. The style of this varies between units, from a detailed 'board round' to walking around the unit handing over each patient at the bedside. Important information regarding the patients' progress throughout the preceding shift as well as areas of concern and plans for the day is communicated. The time taken for the handover chiefly depends on the size of the unit and the dependency of the patients, but in a large ICU it is not unusual for the handover to take over half an hour.

Once the handover is completed, patient reviews will begin (often after a morning coffee). This consists of a full assessment of each patient, reviewing all aspects of their treatment, including a review of the medical history, investigation results, medication charts, fluid and nutritional requirements and physiotherapy requirements. Physical examination using the ABCDE approach, which is familiar to all medical graduates, is a very useful scheme to make sure nothing is omitted until one becomes familiar enough to develop one's own system. The daily review is covered in detail in Chapter 2.

During the daily review, you will be confronted with the vast array of equipment in each bed space. There will be a monitor screen with more sections than you might expect, and each patient may well be connected to a host of syringe drivers and infusion pumps, in addition to a ventilator and other organ support. To the ICU beginner this can be an intimidating sight; however, with time this becomes part of the scenery! The details of this complex equipment are discussed in later chapters, but on your first day there are a few things worth looking at early on. The ICU chart is a repository of useful information. The format can differ but the essential elements remain the same. Routine observations you might expect to see on a ward chart are documented, in general at least hourly, but in addition to this you may well find ventilator parameters, blood gas results, detailed fluid balance monitoring, neurological observations and much more. Much of the information you require for your daily review will come from this chart, and as you get used to where this information is located, you will find the daily reviews considerably easier.

In many ICUs, the daily reviews are carried out by juniors, followed by a consultant-led round. You will be expected to present the patients you have reviewed and, as you gain experience, formulate a plan for these patients. In other units, the daily reviews and ward round are combined into a more detailed consultant round. Once the consultant round is complete, any further jobs can be carried out. The remainder of the day will largely consist of dealing with queries from nurses or other healthcare professionals. Depending on the patient, their 'parent' team may well review the patient on their ward round and contribute to the daily management plans.

Urgent jobs are carried out as the need arises. The on-call medical staff may well be called away to review unwell patients on the ward, and if there are many patients requiring ICU review, more people may have to leave the unit. You will need to be flexible to ensure that all patients in the ICU are reviewed in a timely fashion.

WHO TO ASK FOR HELP

The nurses in the ICU are a vital part of patient care and can make your life very easy. They may well know much of what has happened to a patient even if it is not well documented in the medical notes, and can make your daily reviews quicker. As with many aspects of medicine, when you begin in ICU, they may well know much more than you about their area of expertise. In addition, in ICU, the medical staff are significantly outnumbered by nursing staff, as the nurses look after one to two patients each. Do not be afraid to ask for their advice if you are unsure about something, and if they are unhappy with your plan for their patient, it is well worth reconsidering. It may well be that your plan is appropriate, but often they will have greater insight into how things are usually done in the ICU.

Other trainees can be an invaluable source of help when you are first starting in intensive care. Anaesthetic trainees make up a large part of the trainee workforce, in addition to medical trainees. There may also be trainees on an intensive care medicine training programme, either alone or in conjunction with another specialty. Some ICUs have advanced critical care practitioners, who are often very experienced ICU nurses or other associate healthcare professionals who have undertaken training approved by the Faculty of Intensive Care Medicine (FICM). Their role can vary from trust to trust, but they are qualified to undertake many of the tasks usually associated with ICU doctors. Obviously, the consultants are available for advice in addition to the other team members mentioned, and guidelines require a consultant to be available at all times and to carry out twice-daily ward rounds. Consultant presence is very high in critical care, and the junior medical staff are very well supported by seniors. Do not be afraid to call your consultant; if on call, they will be expecting it!

There are many specialists who are not based in critical care but without whose help the ICU could not work. This includes microbiologists, who may carry out regular ward rounds, pharmacists, who are often heavily involved in intensive care, and physiotherapists, without whose assistance many patients would not leave the unit.

ICU TERMINOLOGY

Unique vocabulary is an aspect of any medical specialty that can be challenging to the newcomer. There are many acronyms and terms specific to intensive care that you may come across in the medical notes or in discussions about the patient. These can seem rather opaque, relating to medication, interventions or conditions associated with the ICU. Many of them will be covered in subsequent chapters, but in particular, advanced respiratory support is an area full of acronyms that you will come across frequently to describe ventilator modes and parameters. In addition, cardiac output monitor results contain many acronyms, many of which remain equally confusing when you discover what they stand for. As you come across these acronyms, do ask for explanations or look them up, as it will deepen your understanding of the specialty.

2

The daily review of a patient

SHONDIPON K. LAHA

This is an important aspect of intensive care. Many of the patients have complex co-morbidities and pathology, and a systematic method of assessing them allows problems to be broken down and a management plan to be instituted.

This review is the backbone of care for the critically ill patient and will be the bulk of your workload. It may appear to be prolonged initially but after practice should become second nature. This allows you to recognise and manage critically ill patients in other environments.

PRIMARY DIAGNOSIS

- Why have they been admitted? (e.g. pneumonia)

BACKGROUND AND PROGRESS

- A summary of past medical history and the history of this admission, followed by what has happened over the course of their intensive care unit (ICU) stay.

ISSUES OVER THE LAST 24 HOURS

- A summary of any problems or improvements since the last review.

RESPIRATORY SYSTEM

- Examination of the respiratory system.
- Are they intubated or do they have a tracheostomy?/What kind of tube is it and what size?
- How are they being ventilated and what are the settings?
- Amount and character of any sputum.
- Oxygen saturation and arterial blood gases.
- When was the last chest X-ray and what did it show?
- Are they on any respiratory medication?

CARDIOVASCULAR SYSTEM

- Palpation of pulses.
- Peripheral oedema extent.
- Capillary refill.
- Blood pressure (including mean arterial pressure).
- Heart rate and rhythm.
- Electrocardiography (ECG).
- Central venous pressure.

- Cardiac output monitoring.
- If they have had an echo done, document the results and when it was performed.
- Any cardiac medication including inotropes, vasopressors and antihypertensives.

RENAL SYSTEM

- Average urine output (mL/hour).
- Total fluid in and out in last 24 hours and overall balance.
- The patient's weight (are they becoming overloaded?).
- Have they needed diuretics in the last 24 hours?
- Have they needed renal replacement therapy in the last 24 hours (i.e. dialysis or filtration)?
- Electrolyte results.

GASTROINTESTINAL SYSTEM

- Are there any abnormalities on examination?
- By what route are they being fed? (nasogastric, TPN, none)
- What kind of feed are they receiving?
- Is it being absorbed?
- At what rate is the feed being given?
- When did they last open their bowels?
- Are they on any gastric medication (prokinetics, laxatives, gastric pH modifying drugs)?
- Liver function test results.

HAEMATOLOGY

- Haemoglobin, platelet and clotting results.
- Have they needed transfusions in the last 24 hours?
- Are they on any anticoagulation medication?

NEUROLOGICAL SYSTEM

- What is their sedation score?
- What is their Glasgow Coma Scale?
- Have there been any episodes of delirium or any recorded scores?
- Neurological examination (pupils, power, tone and reflexes).
- Neurological medication (sedatives, muscle relaxants, anti-epileptics).
- If on a neurosurgical unit, then the intracranial pressure, the amount of drainage from an EVD and whether they needed treatment for neurological problems overnight should be documented.

MICROBIOLOGY

- Any organisms that have been cultured and their sensitivities.
- What antibiotics are they on and for how long?
- The highest temperature in the last 24 hours.
- Their white cell count.

LINES

- What lines have they got in, how long have they been in and is the site clean?

GENERAL

- When were the relatives last spoken to?
- Does the patient have treatment limitations or a 'Do not resuscitate' order?
- Have you reviewed the prescription chart and any recent investigations?

SUMMARY OF ISSUES

- Identify ongoing issues and whether they are improving or worsening.
- Identify new issues over the last 24 hours, and what has been done to remedy them.

TREATMENT PLAN

- List the jobs that needed to be done.

At the end, sign and date your record and make sure your name is legible. A number of units will have electronic patient records whereby much of this information, including username and date, is automatically recorded.

KEY LEARNING POINTS

- The daily systematic review is vital for the continued management of the ICU patient.
- It should cover all the systems and highlight ongoing and new issues.
- Repeated practice should make it easier and give you a framework to assess all critically ill patients.

3

Communication

MARK PUGH AND ROBERT FALLON

WHY IS COMMUNICATION SO IMPORTANT?

Good communication within the multi-disciplinary team and with patients and their relatives is essential to the efficient running of a intensive care unit. In 2015–2016, the NHS received over 198,000 written complaints; just over 10% were related to communication.

Effective communication is essential to the well being of your patient and to your future medical career. It will be assessed on a regular basis throughout your training.

In the intensive care unit, the patient's outcome relies upon good communication within the intensive care multi-disciplinary team, the referring specialty team and other departments within the hospital. The majority of this communication will involve junior members of the clinical team, which means *you*.

WHO WILL I BE COMMUNICATING WITH?

ON THE INTENSIVE CARE UNIT

- The patient and their family/next of kin
- The nurse looking after the patient
- The sister/charge nurse with overall responsibility
- Junior and senior medical colleagues
- Allied health professionals (physiotherapists, dietitian, pharmacists, radiographers, etc.)

IN THE HOSPITAL

- Referring teams, emergency department, anaesthetists
- Other departments (e.g. laboratory staff, radiology, pharmacy)

OUTSIDE THE HOSPITAL

- The patient's general practitioner
- The coroner/police

HOW CAN I COMMUNICATE EFFECTIVELY WITHIN THE MULTI-DISCIPLINARY TEAM?

Effective communication is dependent to a large extent upon mutual respect and trust. It is essential to acknowledge everyone's role within the multi-disciplinary team, and to recognise that patient outcomes depend upon all aspects of care delivery, not just the doctor's role. Remember that you are a small yet essential cog in a large machine.

For some medical practitioners this is a difficult concept to grasp. Some advice for a long and hassle-free career is given below.

ALWAYS

- Introduce yourself to the patient and to the nurse who is looking after them.
- Listen to and acknowledge the concerns of others.
- Explain the reasons for your decisions.
- Admit when you don't know the answer.
- Admit when you are wrong.

NEVER

- Ignore or talk down to patients or members of the multi-disciplinary team.
- 'Blag' or work outside your proven competencies.
- Argue or disagree forcibly with team members in front of patients, relatives or other staff.
- Try to 'score points' within the team.
- Try to hide your mistakes or omissions.

For situations in which you are discussing clinical issues, especially over the telephone with senior medical staff, there is a widely used system to aid communication, the SBAR approach:

- **S**ituation:
    - Identify yourself and the unit you are calling from.
    - Identify the patient and reason for your call.
    - Describe your concern.

- **B**ackground
  - Give the reason and date of the patient's admission.
  - Explain the significant medical history.
  - Give the admission diagnosis, prior procedures, medications, allergies, and laboratory and diagnostic results.
- **A**ssessment:
  - Vital signs.
  - Clinical impressions/concerns.
  - Measures already taken.
- **R**ecommendations:
  - Explain what you need; be specific about what you need and when, e.g. 'I need you to see this patient now' rather than 'I would like you to see this patient soon'.
  - Make suggestions.
  - Clarify expectations, especially if advice is given over the phone. Repeat it back to ensure accuracy.

This system works well, with a few provisos. Before picking up the phone, always make sure that:

- You know the patient and situation well.
- You have carried out a thorough assessment, including examining the patient.
- You have started some even simple measures to improve the situation and asked for appropriate help within the multi-disciplinary team.
- You have a clear idea of what you want to happen.

As with all communication, a concise account of the conversation should be documented in the notes. The recommendations/actions to be taken should be clearly stated. The account should include the date and time (using the 24-hour clock), and a legible signature should be provided, with your name, position and GMC number printed clearly underneath. Remember to record whom you spoke to. The notes remain a legal document and are your best defence should matters be challenged at a later date.

HOW CAN I COMMUNICATE EFFECTIVELY WITH PATIENTS AND RELATIVES?

It is important to remember that not all patients in intensive care are unconscious, even those who may be on some form of sedation.

Always

- Introduce yourself to the patient as though they can hear you (they often can, despite appearances).
- Explain what you are about to do before performing an examination or procedure.
- Treat the patient with respect and dignity.
- Be positive.

Never

- Assume the patient is unconscious.
- Make comments about the patient's prognosis or progress (unless they are positive) within earshot.
- Make disparaging or hurtful comments.
- Gossip or talk about other patients within earshot.

When major decisions about treatment are made, remember to involve the patient directly wherever possible. A lack of capacity does not mean that you should not attempt to explain what is happening and why.

HOW DO I BREAK BAD NEWS?

Most UK doctors undergo extensive training as undergraduates in communication skills, including how to break bad news. However, this does not make you an expert.

Ideally, the most senior clinical available should lead conversations about withdrawing and withholding treatment, preferably in the daytime when there is plenty of support for patients and their relatives are immediately available.

Whenever the opportunity arises, observe others breaking bad news. You will see both good and bad ways of going about it, and be able to decide what works best for you in these situations. When breaking bad news for the first time, take someone senior with you for moral support.

By far the best model approach for breaking bad news was described by Buckman. Although primarily designed for use by oncologists, it is easily adaptable for intensive care. The approach is summarised below.

Spikes model

- Setting, listening skills
- Patient's/relatives' perceptions
- Invite patient/relative to share information
- Knowledge transmission
- Explore emotions and empathise
- Summarise and strategise

Remember that in the case of conscious patients you should always attempt to talk with the patient first. Some patients may not wish to discuss major issues, but you should always attempt to do so, and document that you have attempted. Before speaking to the relatives of a conscious patient, first ensure that the patient is happy for you to do so.

The setting is important. Every unit should have an interview room of sufficient size to allow these conversations to occur away from the bedside and in privacy.

The model works well because it ensures that the majority of the process is concentrated on you listening to the patient's or relative's perceptions and fears, rather than being focused on the doctor giving information and/or making decisions. Some more advice for a better outcome is given below.

Always

- Ensure that you know the patient and their diagnosis and prognosis well.
- Take the nurse who is looking after the patient with you.
- Introduce yourself and any other members of the team who are present, and ask the family to introduce themselves (you would not want to mistake a patient's wife for their mother, or vice versa).
- Establish the patient's known wishes.
- Keep matters simple and avoid the use of jargon.
- Take your time. If a family is struggling to understand and come to terms with what you are saying, back off and arrange to speak to them again later.
- Use clear terms (e.g. 'die', 'futile').
- Document clearly the outcome of the meeting.

NEVER

- Begin a conversation without full knowledge of the situation.
- Rush.
- Be ambitious.
- Blame other teams or specialties for a poor outcome.
- Break a patient's confidence.

CONCLUSION

Effective communication can be easily achieved if you remember to respect and value those around you. Remember to treat people as you would wish to be treated yourself and you won't go far wrong.

FURTHER READING

Buckman, Rob. *How to Break Bad News, A Guide for Healthcare Professionals.* Baltimore: Johns Hopkins University Press, 1992.

Health and Social Care Information Centre. *Data on Written Complaints in the NHS 2015-16.* Leeds: Workforce and Facilities Team, Health and Social Care Information Centre, 2016.

NHS Institute for Innovation and Improvement. *Safer Care. SBAR – Situation-Background-Assessment-Recommendation.* Warwick: NHS Institute for Innovation and Improvement. 2010.

4

Capacity and consent

ANGELA DAY AND MICHAEL ELLIOT

It is 2 am and you are bleeped by the nurses about the patient in Bed 3. He is a 65-year-old man, being treated for sepsis with antibiotics and noradrenaline. He is intermittently confused and pulling at his lines. He has just pulled out his arterial line and is refusing to allow it to be re-sited. The nurses are requesting your help.

Similar situations are not uncommon in critical care, and knowledge of capacity and consent is vital to ensure you are providing treatment within General Medical Council (GMC) guidelines and the law.

CONSENT

Consent is the legal agreement to an intervention and can be either implied, explicit or presumed.

- **Implied consent** – the patient makes an action to allow a proposed intervention (e.g. they hold out their arm when asked for a blood sample).
- **Explicit consent** – an intervention is discussed with the patient and they agree with the intervention. The agreement can be verbal or written. Whilst there is no legal difference in the validity of these, it is easier to prove consent if it is written. Verbal consent for a procedure should be documented in the patient's notes.
- **Presumed consent** – this applies when a patient does not have capacity to consent to the intervention proposed. It is based upon the premise that they would consent if they did have capacity, and the intervention is considered to be in their best interest.

Without the permission of the patient, many interventions we perform are illegal, constituting battery or assault.

- **Battery** is the unlawful application of physical force to another.
- **Assault** is an attempt to commit battery or an act which may cause fear of imminent battery.

CAPACITY

For a patient to give valid consent, they must have the **capacity** to make the decision being asked of them. Patients must always be assumed to have capacity, unless it has been established that they do not. To assess capacity, you should ascertain whether

1. The patient **understands** and **believes** the information given about the proposed action.
2. They are able to **retain** this information.
3. They are able to **weigh up** the information given in order to reach a decision.
4. They are able to **communicate** their decision.

Patients with capacity are free to accept or refuse any treatment that is offered. A seemingly unwise or irrational decision does not denote lack of capacity. If there is any doubt whether the patient has capacity, seek a second opinion.

Capacity relates to the decision at hand; a patient may be perfectly able to agree to provide a blood sample, but lack the capacity to consent to major surgery. Patients must be given as much support as they require to help them make their own decisions where possible. When a patient lacks capacity, it is important to identify the cause – anything reversible should be treated. It should also be considered whether the decision could wait for the patient to regain capacity, if that is likely to occur.

LACK OF CAPACITY

Some patients make arrangements to allow for consent to decisions to be made at a time when they lack capacity. This can be done in two ways:

- An **advance directive** is a legal document signed and witnessed by the patient while they had capacity. It outlines what interventions they would and would not consent to. This has the same legal standing as a decision made by a patient with capacity. However, it must be specific to the situation at hand, which can be difficult to verify in an emergency. If in doubt, seek senior advice.
- A person with **lasting power of attorney (health and welfare)** is someone appointed by the patient, at a time when they had capacity, authorised to make decisions on their behalf. Again, this has the same standing as the patient's own decision.

In the absence of either of these, treatment for a patient lacking capacity should proceed upon what is deemed to be in their best interest. Determining this is not always straightforward. First, it is vital to try to identify what the patient's wishes were likely to have been; this can be done by consulting relatives, friends or carers. If there is nobody to represent their view, a request to appoint an Independent Mental Capacity Advocate (IMCA) should be made. The final decision is usually made by the medical team caring for the patient, but with respect for their wishes. In the event of any disagreement about the patient's best interests, senior advice should be sought. When uncertainty persists, occasionally the Court of Protection is asked for a ruling.

DEPRIVATION OF LIBERTY SAFEGUARDS

Deprivation of Liberty Safeguards (DoLS) was added to the Mental Capacity Act in 2007, in order to protect vulnerable adults from being unlawfully deprived of their liberty. If they are placed in a situation where they are unable to leave should they wish to, patients admitted to the hospital are being deprived of their liberty. This has created uncertainty in recent years, as many patients in critical care would not be free to leave. The most recent Department of Health guidance states that for DoLS to apply, the patient's lack of capacity should be due to a mental disorder (as defined within the Mental Health Act). Thus, patients sedated for treatment of a physical illness do not fall within the framework of DoLS. The Court of Appeal (2017) has pronounced that life-saving treatment does not generally constitute a deprivation of liberty.

RESTRAINT

Sometimes it is necessary to restrain a patient, either physically or chemically, to prevent them from harming themselves or others. This should only be done if they lack capacity. Any such actions should be with the intent of preventing harm, and proportionate to the severity of harm that might occur. It is good practice to try persuasion before embarking upon restraint.

MENTAL HEALTH ACT 1983

The Mental Health Act sets out situations in which a patient may be detained for assessment and treatment of mental health disorders without their consent. This does not allow treatment of any physical disorder without consent. However, the patient's mental condition may mean that they do not have capacity to consent to physical treatment. In this situation, they should be treated in their best interests as previously described.

CHILDREN

Whilst this area can be complex, the principles are as follows:

- Young people aged 16–17 years
  - In Scotland, the legal age of capacity is 16.

- In other UK jurisdictions, a person who has reached the age of 16 is presumed to have the same capacity as an adult to consent to treatment.
  - You should not reveal information about these patients to their parents without the patient's consent.
- Children under 16 years
  - A child under the age of 16 may have capacity. The legal test is 'Gillick competence'. This states that if the child understands the consequences of a decision, they have capacity.
  - It is generally best practice to obtain parental assent. However, if a Gillick competent child insists upon confidentiality, this should be respected.
  - A person with parental responsibility can always consent for a child under 16, even if the child is Gillick competent.
- Withholding consent
  - If the child is not Gillick competent, the parents can consent on behalf of the child, even if the child refuses treatment.
  - If a child is competent, the law around a parent overriding the child's refusal is complex. Careful consideration should be given to whether overriding the child's refusal is in their best interest. If there were any doubt, it would be wise to seek a second opinion. In Scotland, parents cannot override refusal of consent by a competent child.
- Treatment in an emergency
  - In an emergency, if a person with parental responsibility is not available to consent for treatment, the doctor should act in accordance with the child's best interests. This should be discussed with a senior doctor and clearly documented.

ANSWER TO CLINICAL SCENARIO

- You need to assess the patient's capacity – it seems unlikely that he has capacity, and could be confused because of his infection.
- Initially, you should attempt to persuade him to allow the arterial line to be re-sited.
- Some level of chemical and/or physical restraint may be necessary to allow treatment to proceed in his best interests. This should be proportionate and as minimally restrictive as possible. A sedative or small dose

of antipsychotic would be a sensible choice. If he continues to pull at his lines, you may consider whether he needs mittens to prevent further loss of lines.

KEY LEARNING POINTS

- Mentally competent adults are free to consent or withhold consent for treatment, even if their decision seems unwise.
- Patients must be assumed to have mental capacity unless proven otherwise.
- For patients lacking capacity, and in the absence of a lasting power of attorney, treatment must be decided by staff in the patient's best interests.
- DoLS are not generally relevant for life-saving treatment.

FURTHER READING

Department of Constitutional Affairs. *Mental Capacity Act 2005: Code of Practice*. London: The Stationery Office, 2007. https://www.gov.uk /government/uploads/system/uploads/attachment_data/file/497253 /Mental-capacity-act-code-of-practice.pdf (accessed 13 February 2017).

Department of Health. *Mental Health Act 1983: Code of Practice*. London: The Stationery Office, 2015. https://www.gov.uk/government/uploads /system/uploads/attachment_data/file/435512/MHA_Code_of _Practice.PDF (accessed 13 February 2017).

General Medical Council. *0–18 years: Guidance for all Doctors*. London: General Medical Council, 2007. http://www.gmc-uk.org/0_18_years _English_1015.pdf_48903188.pdf (accessed 13 February 2017).

General Medical Council. *Consent—Patients and Doctors Making Decisions Together*. London: General Medical Council, 2008. http://www.gmc-uk.org /Consent_English_1015.pdf_48903482.pdf (accessed 13 February 2017).

5

FOAMed and social media as an aid to education in intensive care

JONATHAN DOWNHAM

> *'But I was listening to a podcast last night when they said this was the new way of doing this procedure...'*

'Social Media: Websites and applications that enable users to create and share content or to participate in social networking'.

English Oxford Living Dictionaries

The way we learn and keep up to date has changed dramatically over the last 10–15 years. With advances in processing power and increasingly fast download speeds across the internet, we now have many more options at our disposal when we seek out information.

The internet, however, is only the medium by which this information is being brought to us. Via this medium, we now have access to video, audio and the written word, all of which can be updated and disseminated almost as quickly as it can be filmed, said or written. In the critical care and emergency medicine spheres, the numbers are expanding all the time; as of November 2013, 141 blogs and 42 podcasts were identified on 183 websites. It can only be assumed that this number will continue to grow.

The advent of 'social media', which can be defined as 'websites and applications that enable users to create and share content or to participate in social networking', has ensured that this information can be spread far more quickly than in the past, via Twitter, Facebook, YouTube, LinkedIn and many others.

FREE OPEN ACCESS MEDICAL EDUCATION (FOAMed)

FOAMed is a movement that has grown alongside the social media channels that support it. The title itself is self-explanatory as to what it entails, but it is important to say that FOAMed itself is also a concept with a number of tenets that makes it work so well.

It is about sharing medical education resources, wherever they may be found. Many of the sharers of the resources are also the creators, but many others are just sign posting online resources they have found to be useful. Much of this information is of high quality and this is certainly embedded within the FOAMed concept.

FOAMed is also about the interaction that is generated by the sharing of the resources found. This interaction can lead to many valuable conversations enabling further refinement of some of the information and resources shared.

Creators of resources are positively encouraging of its reuse, without charge, but preferably with attribution for the work that has gone into it. It should be remembered that although the word 'free' is in the title, someone has generally gone to some trouble to make the blog/webpage/video/podcast/ infographic. Recognising that hard work is important, and vital, to ensure that the FOAMed concept continues to thrive.

TWITTER

There is now a continual cascade of information via the internet, which could affect the way we practise. One way to keep up to date with this wealth of information is via Twitter.

Twitter, which has been central to the FOAMed movement, is great for sharing links and other resources and the use of its hashtag will supply the user with a wealth of information on a regular basis.

Like many of the other social platforms, Twitter is free to set up and use, and one can follow anyone else to see what they have to say. The common misconception amongst those who do not use this platform is that only trivia is normally exchanged. If one follows the right people, this is very far from the truth.

I am often asked by new users who they should follow. My instant reply to this is not who, but what. If you are interested in sepsis, for example, then this is the subject you should pursue and this is where the hashtag comes into its own.

The experienced user, when tweeting something of interest, will add a hashtag to that message – #sepsis for example. If one then searches Twitter using #sepsis, that message – and any other with the same hashtag – will appear in the results. As well as allowing a quick and simple search, this will also then allow the user to go and follow any or all of those Twitter users who have shown an interest in sepsis.

Using this mechanism for any area of interest will quickly allow you to connect with like-minded users.

The messages sent via Twitter are limited to 280 characters (140 characters until October 2017). Some may see this as a limitation; however, it should be seen as strength as Twitter is used as a sign-posting mechanism to other resources, rather than a series of long posts on the platform itself. Images can also be added to the messages, which do not take away from the character count. These images can be used to reinforce the point of the message, add to the information contained in it or simply help catch the user's eye as they scroll through their stream.

When using Twitter, it is important to remember a number of things. First, do not be anonymous. The interactivity thrives because there are real people on there sharing their experiences, resources and opinions. If necessary, have separate accounts to keep professional and personal lives separate. Second, try to be as active as possible. This will ensure that others will follow you and share resources with you. I promise you will develop relationships with other professionals that you might never meet otherwise. Lastly, be generous with your tweets. By this I mean do not hesitate to let others know about valuable resources you have made or discovered, and retweet the work of others. They will appreciate it and may do the same for your hard work one day.

Podcasts

Podcasts started to appear around 2004 and, in 2005, Apple added podcasting to its iTunes software making them easier to access. If you think they are a fairly minor phenomenon that is not growing, think again:

- In 2007, Ricky Gervais set a record for the most downloaded podcasts in a month – over 260,000.
- In 2011, Adam Carolla became a Guinness World Records holder after his podcast received over 59 million downloads over the previous two years.
- In 2013, Apple announced 1 billion podcast subscribers.
- In 2015, President Obama was interviewed on a podcast.

Accessing podcasts is now far easier than in previous years. With the recent development in smart phones, one can now set the episodes to download automatically as they are released. There are apps available such as Pocketcasts, Overcast and Podcast Republic, which will all help automate and organise your library, meaning that the reliance on iTunes is not necessary.

Podcasts cover a huge range of subjects but there are many discussing the issues around Critical Care and Emergency Medicine. They range in length from about 15 minutes to an hour and are released anywhere between weekly to once or twice a year.

There are a number of benefits to podcasts:

- Unlike video learning, they do not require you to sit in front of a screen devoting all your time to them. Many people listen to them whilst doing other activities such as running, driving or walking the dog. Listening whilst driving can be considered an efficient use of otherwise 'wasted' time.
- They can be listened to in bite-sized chunks and repeatedly if needed. Very often if I do not understand something well, I will listen to the same podcast several times.
- Many episodes can be stored at once. This ensures that you can be carrying around a wealth of information with you to access at your leisure.
- Because the podcast can be downloaded as soon as it is published, it can be considered very up to date.

Blogs/websites

Possibly one of the best known in this category is *Life in the Fast Lane*, which is a collaborative website led by Chris Nickson, a doctor in Australia.

In addition to being a huge repository of many things to do with critical care and emergency medicine, it is also the host site for the weekly roundup from around the web for all things FOAMed. This site also has great connections with its Twitter feed from where you can see what is new on the site.

There are many other blogs and websites from around the world now offering various perspectives from diverse practitioners across the specialties.

Probably the easiest way to find them is to use *Life in the Fast Lane's* resource: Emergency Medicine and Critical Care Database. On this page they have listed all the websites and blogs they know of and are making efforts to keep this up to date.

NOT ALL THAT GLITTERS IS GOLD

Perhaps a final note should be to acknowledge that FOAMed is not scientific research but rather a way of disseminating knowledge that can then become part of a thread and discussed by many across the globe. It is also, like all of the printed literature, an adjunct to bedside learning and an aid to mentoring that will help produce a better practitioner.

The user also needs to be careful when using FOAMed. An article can be written and posted by anyone so one should always be aware of the potential shortcomings of such a process. Whilst there is a lot of peer review occurring because of the very nature of social media, it does not necessarily follow that every item you read should be accepted as current practice/thinking. Continue to talk to your senior, more experienced colleagues and learn from them.

However, it is hoped that with the on-going discussions by many experienced and knowledgeable practitioners that the bubbles will always rise to the top!

KEY LEARNING POINTS

- FOAMed and social media can be a valuable free resource.
- Useful resources include Twitter, podcasts and blogs.
- Be wary of using FOAMed as it is not scientific research but a way of disseminating knowledge that can be produced by anyone.

FURTHER READING

Websites/blogs

Critical Care Reviews (www.criticalcarereviews.com)
EMCrit (http://emcrit.org)
ICM Case Summaries (http://icmcasesummaries.com)
Life in the Fast Lane (http://lifeinthefastlane.com)
PHARM: Prehospital and Retrieval Medicine (http://prehospitalmed.com)

Podcasts

SMACC: Social Media and Critical Care (http://smacc2013.libsyn.com)
St Emlyns (www.stemlynspodcast.org)
The Bottom Line (www.thebottomline.org.uk/podcasts)

6

Research in intensive care

CATRIONA FRANKLING AND GAVIN PERKINS

WHY IS RESEARCH IMPORTANT?

Research in the critical care setting can lead to improvement in the quality of patient care through evidence-based medicine. For instance, research into acute respiratory distress syndrome (ARDS) has led to the development of lung-protective strategies that have decreased the incidence of lung injury in ventilated patients. Blood glucose is no longer as tightly controlled as it used to be in the intensive care unit (ICU) after research demonstrated the detrimental effects of strict blood glucose control. Both of these areas of research have benefitted ICU patients.

COMMON TYPES OF RESEARCH IN ICU

TRANSLATIONAL SCIENCE

This type of research aims to bridge the gap between laboratory research and applied science. In medicine, this involves the application of in vitro studies to clinical practice. Translational medicine requires a multidisciplinary approach to ensure that both laboratory and clinical researchers work towards the same research goals, resulting in bench-side studies that are relevant to patients.

EARLY PHASE CLINICAL STUDIES

This is the first step in testing a new treatment that has been developed in the laboratory. It may involve testing very low sub-therapeutic doses of a drug in patients to gather information about how the drug is distributed and metabolised in the body. It may also collect data on whether the drug affects the correct molecular target. These types of studies can ensure that it is worth investing the time and funding to pursue a new drug therapy, and therefore help determine whether larger studies on a new drug are appropriate.

OBSERVATIONAL STUDIES

These studies do not involve an intervention or exposure assigned by the study investigators. There are different types, such as cohort studies, and cross-sectional studies. The data from these types of studies will be subject to bias because the researcher cannot control which patients are exposed to the treatment or disease that they are studying. An example of an observational study in ICU would be the collection of data on lung ventilation settings and mortality. This can be used to assess whether patients whose ventilator settings adhered to a lung protective strategy had lower mortality rates than patients who did not have lung protective ventilation. There is the risk of confounding in this type of study, as the two groups may be dissimilar in ways other than the type of lung ventilation. It is possible to apply statistical methods to attempt to reduce bias. Propensity score matching is a statistical method that aims to reduce bias due to confounding variables. It aims to make the intervention and non-intervention groups more comparable. However, bias will still be a risk, as it cannot account for all possible variables.

RANDOMISED CONTROLLED TRIALS (RCTs)

This is a type of experimental study. Patients enrolled into randomised controlled trials will be randomly allocated either to the group receiving the intervention being studied, or to the group receiving current standard medical treatment (or placebo). The other type of experimental study is called non-randomised. Non-randomised studies are at risk of allocation bias and confounding. Randomisation avoids allocation bias and should result in similar baseline characteristics in each study group, therefore avoiding confounding. An example of an RCT is the BALTI-2 trial. Patients with ARDS were randomised to receive either an intravenous infusion of salbutamol or placebo (0.9% sodium chloride infusion). This study demonstrated that salbutamol infusion was unlikely to be beneficial in ARDS and may make outcomes worse. Even studies, such as this, that have negative results are useful, as these findings will mean that future patients will not be given potentially harmful treatment. This type of study is an effectiveness (pragmatic) trial and looks at how beneficial an intervention is in 'real world' clinical settings. In contrast, efficacy (explanatory) trials look at whether an intervention produces the expected result under ideal circumstances. The BALTI-1 trial was an efficacy trial, which led to the BALTI-2 trial. The BALTI-1 trial found that there was in-vivo evidence of reduced alveolar capillary permeability in patients treated with salbutamol. This led to the effectiveness BALTI-2 trial, which in turn showed that the positive results found in BALTI-1 did not translate to 'real world' improvements in patient outcomes.

PRACTICAL ASPECTS OF RESEARCH IN ICU

WHO CARRIES OUT THE RESEARCH?

This will vary depending on the ICU. Some ICUs that are heavily involved in research will have a dedicated team of research nurses and doctors who will manage several research projects at any one time. The research nurses will visit ICU daily to recruit patients and follow up on any patients already enrolled into a study. However, many ICUs will not have any dedicated research nurses and instead research may be managed by a full-time clinical consultant alongside their other roles and responsibilities.

CONSENT

Most ICU patients will lack capacity to consent to research. Capacity requires a patient to understand the information given to them, retain the information, and convey a decision to those treating them. Other areas of their medical treatment will be decided based on what is in the patient's best interest. However, when it comes to research, it is difficult to decide whether it is in their best interest. Research is conducted because we do not know what the best treatment or management of a condition is. Therefore, any research carried out may not benefit the patient involved in the research. This means that the consent process for research is different than for standard medical treatment, and is tightly governed to ensure vulnerable patients are protected. To find out more about the consent process in research, especially for patients who lack capacity to consent, you can undertake training in Good Clinical Practice (GCP). GCP training ensures all research is carried out to the highest ethical, scientific and practical standards. It is mandatory for staff conducting research, but is also beneficial to anyone working in ICU who will be exposed to research.

ETHICAL ASPECTS OF RESEARCH IN ICU

As already discussed, ICU patients are often unable to consent to involvement in research, yet they are still enrolled into studies. Their involvement in a study may not benefit the patient in any way, and could even potentially result in harm. To protect patients from potential harm from research, all studies will go through an ethics committee for approval before they can be started. These committees will consider the potential harms and benefits for the patients involved in the study, as well as the potential benefit to future patients from the results of the study. Ethics committees give much thought and consideration to all research projects involving patients, with strict rules and regulations to protect research participants.

If you plan to conduct research, then you must apply for ethical approval for your study through the Health Research Authority.

HOW TO GET INVOLVED IN RESEARCH IN ICU

This can range from superficial involvement in data collection, to becoming part of a research team.

At the simplest level, all doctors in ICU will be involved in research, as data collection for research will record data from the patient's notes. It is important to ensure that notes are written clearly and accurately. For example, if the admission notes omit a patient's chronic renal failure, this will not only potentially affect the patient's care but will also lead to inaccurate data collection for audit and research.

If you would like to become more involved in research, speak to the nurse or doctor leading research in your ICU and ask how you can help. There may be a small project you can complete, or you may be able to help with part of a larger project. If you have any ideas, then speak to the research team or your supervising consultant; they may be able to help you put your idea into fruition. Remember though that research takes time, and projects will require ethical approval before commencement, so you may not be able to see your project through to the end.

If you are interested in a career in research, there are several different ways to enter the career path for research. You can find out more via the National Institute for Health Research (NIHR) website. Many regions will offer clinical research posts between 6 to 24 months long. It is also possible to combine clinical training with academic pursuits through foundation academic training, clinical fellow and clinical lecturer posts. To find out what is available in your area, speak to doctors currently involved in research, check the career pages of the *British Medical Journal* and speak to your supervisor.

KEY LEARNING POINTS

- Everyone who works in ICU will be involved in research in some way.
- Without research, patient care cannot be evidence-based and potentially harmful treatments may be given to patients.
- Research in ICU involves patients who lack capacity to consent. There are strict rules governing this to protect patients.

FURTHER READING

Camporota, Luigi, and Nicholas Hart. "Lung Protective Ventilation." *The BMJ*, 344 (2012): e2491.

National Institute for Health Research. *NIHR Trainees Coordinating Centre.* http://www.nihr.ac.uk/about-us/how-we-are-managed/managing-centres/about-the-trainees-coordinating-centre.htm (accessed 31 January 2017).

NICE-SUGAR Study Investigators. "Intensive versus Conventional Glucose Control in Critically Ill Patients." *New England Journal of Medicine* 360, no. 13 (March 2009): 1283–1297.

Perkins, Gavin D., Fang Gao, and David R. Thickett. "In Vivo and In Vitro Effects of Salbutamol on Alveolar Epithelial Repair in Acute Lung Injury." *Thorax* 63, no. 3 (2008): 215–220.

Smith, Fang Gao, Gavin D. Perkins, Simon Gates, Duncan Young, Daniel F. McAuley, William Tunnicliffe, Zahid Khan, Sarah E. Lamb, for the BALTI-2 Study Investigators. "Effect of Intravenous ß-2 Agonist Treatment on Clinical Outcomes in Acute Respiratory Distress Syndrome (BALTI-2): A Multicentre, Randomised Controlled Trial." *Lancet* 379, no. 9812 (21 January 2012): 229–235.

7

Stress and burnout in intensive care medicine: Looking after yourself

OLUSEGUN OLUSANYA AND ADRIAN WONG

You are the doctor working on a busy ICU in a tertiary referral hospital. It has been a busy day. The unit is full (again) and there have been a number of referrals from the ward and emergency department that all require intensive care input. The other members of your team have been working hard and without a break. You've been feeling under the weather recently but have still come into work. The constant demands for your attention and advice have made you irritable and you are aware that you've been short and abrupt to colleagues. You begin to question if all this is worth it.

WHAT IS 'BURNOUT'?

The term 'burnout' describes the collection of symptoms and signs, both physical and psychological, experienced by individuals due to their work. It is defined as the condition where professionals 'lose all concerns, all emotional feeling for the people they work with, and come to treat them in a detached or even dehumanised way'. Individuals often feel a sense of emotional exhaustion, indifference, depersonalisation and a lack of desire for personal achievement.

HOW COMMON IS BURNOUT?

Intensive care medicine is well recognised to place high demands (physical and emotional) and considerable levels of stress on practitioners. It is therefore unsurprising that the incidence of burnout and self-harm/suicide is high. A recent survey from the United States suggests a prevalence of 55% amongst critical care physicians, the highest in surveyed medical specialties.

WHO GETS BURNOUT?

Various factors (individual, environmental and organisational) contribute to the risk of developing burnout.

INDIVIDUAL FACTORS

- Age under 55
- Female gender
- Social isolation
- Dysfunctional coping strategies
- Some personality traits

ORGANISATIONAL/WORK-RELATED FACTORS

- Work–life imbalance
- A sense of lacking control
- Unclear job expectations
- Workplace/colleague dysfunction

WHAT ARE THE SIGNS OF BURNOUT?

The clinical symptoms and signs of burnout are often non-specific and can include depression, irritability, insomnia, tiredness and anger. The hallmark of burnout is the triad of

- Emotional exhaustion
- Depersonalisation
- Sense of low personal accomplishment

WHAT ARE THE EFFECTS OF BURNOUT?

Burnout negatively affects the individual, other members of the team and the organisation, and can result in the following:

- Psychological morbidity – depression, anxiety, post-traumatic stress disorder and suicidal behaviour
- Physical morbidity – high blood pressure, fatigue, body aches, reduced concentration and immunosuppression
- Performance and organisational problems – reduced quality of patient care, costs related to absenteeism and high turnover of staff

HOW IS BURNOUT DIAGNOSED?

The tool most widely used to diagnose burnout is the Maslach Burnout Inventory (MBI); this questionnaire consists of 22 items where the responders are asked to indicate the frequency at which they experience certain feelings with regard to their work. Other tools used include the Copenhagen Burnout Inventory and the Oldenburg Burnout Inventory.

ARE THERE ANY TREATMENTS FOR BURNOUT?

A multitude of options exist. Current evidence suggests a two-pronged approach for managing burnout, targeted at both the individual and the organisation. The table below summarises a number of treatment strategies.

Intervention	Aim	Example
ICU organisation	Optimise intensivists' work schedule	Weekend respite Shift models
	Improve work environment	Improved design, natural lighting, well-designed relaxation spaces, comfortable on-call rooms
	Change team composition	Changing theatre lists, 'buddy' systems
	Team-building and job rotation	Planned sabbaticals, varied job plans
	Improving work connectedness and psychological safety	Meeting team members socially, 'fun' events, Schwartz rounds
	Improving sense of value at work	Recognising excellence – 'employee of the month' schemes, excellence meetings
Individual - practical	Educational programme	Well-being seminars
	Communication skills	Non-violent communication, empathic listening
	Relaxation exercise	Yoga, tai chi
	Mindfulness	Mindfulness-based stress reduction courses, online courses, apps
	Physical exercise	Running, joining a gym
	Hobbies	Art, music, reading

Individual - personal	Personality and coping	Emotional intelligence training
	Social support	Arranging regular meet-ups with friends, joining new groups, prioritising family time
	Counselling	Formal psychotherapy, informal through a mentor/friend

I AM FEELING BURNT OUT. WHAT SHOULD I DO?

Anyone who is experiencing symptoms should receive expert help. All doctors should be registered with a general practitioner (GP) who will provide a knowledgeable base from which to seek further assistance. Occupational Health departments are also an excellent initial port of call, and handle all enquiries confidentially. There is no legal obligation for a struggling doctor to inform the General Medical Council.

There are also specialist doctor counselling services available from the British Medical Association and the Royal Medical Benevolent Fund. A nationwide service for GPs is being rolled out, with other specialties almost certain to follow.

CAN BURNOUT BE PREVENTED?

This is an ongoing area of research. It has been suggested that the current manner in which medical practitioners are trained, and the environment in which we practice, makes burnout inevitable. However, many practitioners do not burn out and maintain successful careers for considerable periods of time. Recent studies on individuals who thrive have identified some common themes:

- They experience, or seek out, positive emotions and experience.
- They engage with their work and life.

- They maintain good relationships with friends and family.
- They find meaning in the things they do.
- They seek out and note their accomplishments.

It may be that by combining a focus on such skills, while simultaneously improving working conditions, burnout rates can be improved in the future.

WHAT ABOUT OUR CASE? AN IDEALISED OUTCOME

You work with a kind and compassionate team. A couple of your colleagues notice your mental state, and take you aside for a break. Through their non-judgemental support, you start to recognise that you've been very stressed, sleeping poorly, and have had several bouts of illness within the last few months. You've been increasingly isolated from your friends and family, having missed several important social events – sometimes because of work, but other times because you've just been too tired. Hobbies and exercise have faded into a distant memory.

With your colleagues' encouragement, you make an appointment with the occupational health department where you have a confidential discussion with a doctor. A burnout inventory is performed and you score highly.

An action plan for the next few months is formulated. It is recommended that you have a much-needed two-week break, during which you receive an initial assessment with a clinical psychologist. Your family provides much-needed support at home and you begin to reconnect with some of your previous hobbies and exercises, including yoga and meditation. Quiet periods of reflection and meditation help you to relax.

It is recommended that you would benefit from mindfulness training, cognitive behavioural therapy, and a reduction in your working hours for a few months. While you initially cringe at the idea, preferring to be a 'super doc' and to just 'man up', your doctor and psychologist are insistent. They help you to realise that you cannot pour out of an empty cup, and you just need some time to refill your resources.

Six months later, with continuing support from family and colleagues, you are thriving. You have rediscovered your passion for medicine, and feel that you have grown through your painful experience of a burnout.

KEY LEARNING POINTS

- Burnout is a life-altering syndrome characterised by depersonalisation, emotional exhaustion and a loss of sense of achievement. Left unchecked it can lead to reduced productivity, work absences, and at worst mental illness and suicide. The stresses and prolonged hours in intensive care make us particularly vulnerable.
- Many strategies can be employed to mitigate its effect. Maintaining a strong social network, being physically active, practicing mindfulness, continual learning and maintaining a sense of value all promote resilience. Workplace strategies, such as sabbaticals and work control, may be more effective than individual strategies, or at least synergistic.
- There is also help available for those experiencing symptoms and in distress, both locally and nationally. In the future, many of these strategies will be built into our medical training and will be natural parts of a functioning work environment.

FURTHER READING

Drummond, Dike. *Stop Physician Burnout: What to Do When Working Harder Isn't Working*. Collinsville: Heritage Press Publications. https://www.amazon.com/Stop-Physician-Burnout-Working-Harder/dp/1937660346 (accessed 13 February 2017).

Montgomery, Anthony. "The Inevitability of Physician Burnout." *Burnout Research* 1, no. 1 (June 2014): 50–56. http://www.sciencedirect.com/science/article/pii/S2213058614000084 (accessed 13 February 2017).

Moss, Marc, Vicki S. Good, David Gozal, Ruth Kleinpell, and Curtis N. Sessler. "An Official Critical Care Societies Collaborative Statement – Burnout Syndrome in Critical Care Health-Care Professionals: A Call for Action." *Chest* 150, no. 1 (July 2016): 17–26. https://www.ncbi.nlm.nih.gov/pubmed/27396776 (accessed 13 February 2017).

Public Health England. *Interventions to Prevent Burnout in High Risk Individuals: Evidence Review*. London: Public Health England, 2016. https://www.gov.uk/government/publications/interventions-to-prevent-burnout-in-high-risk-individuals-evidence-review (accessed 13 February 2017).

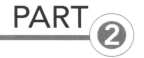

PART 2

STAFFING ON THE INTENSIVE CARE UNIT
The multidisciplinary team

While working in intensive care, you will work closely with a number of different healthcare professionals. This section is an attempt to help you understand how different professions can help critically unwell patients.

The intensive care nurse

GAVIN DENTON

Critical care nurses are typically some of the most highly trained nurses in any given hospital. Although critical care is a highly technical area, basic nursing is still the foundation of the care that a service provides. At one end of the spectrum, the nursing staff will provide oral hygiene for the mechanically ventilated patient to maintain comfort, dental hygiene and reduce the risk from ventilator-associated pneumonia. At the other end of the spectrum, and for the same patient, they may also be responsible for the management of multiple organ failure support such as dialysis or extra-corporeal membrane oxygenation. Nurses also form the linchpin of communication between the multi-disciplinary team (MDT) and family, providing family-centred care. The role of critical care nurses in the UK is very different from that of the United States of America model, where the MDT is larger and different individuals provide various aspects of care. In the UK, all drugs are prepared and administered by the nursing staff, generally perfusionists are absent and extra-corporeal systems are often set up and run by nurses. There are no respiratory therapists to manage non-invasive and invasive ventilation; all of this is the purview of the critical care nurse.

The nurse-to-patient ratio is a vital component of the delivery of critical care, and reflects how broad the role of a critical care nurse is. Level three patients, those receiving mechanical ventilation and multi-system support, are typically provided one-to-one nursing. Level two patients (high dependency level) are usually nursed on a two-to-one ratio.

WHAT TRAINING DO CRITICAL CARE NURSES HAVE?

Critical care nurses are registered adult nurses and have been through three years of basic training. There is no minimum experience required post-registration to work in critical care, although experience is frequently expected. A nurse new to critical care will often receive around six weeks of supernumerary one-to-one mentorship before caring for patients relatively unsupervised. From this point on, individual hospitals will have development programs to train new staff in delivering care and managing machines for different organ support and pathology. Typically, critical care nurses will have to fulfil an extensive competency framework, which incorporates technical aspects of organ support, sub-specialty care and psychosocial aspects.

Sisters or charge nurses have additional training and experience. To attain a junior sister/charge nurse post, staff are usually expected to have a degree-level diploma in critical care nursing and will have at least three years' experience in critical care.

Over the last 10–15 years, critical care nursing has expanded its role by the provision of services in the wider hospital: 'critical care without walls'. Critical care outreach teams often form part of resuscitation and emergency response teams on general wards. These teams fit within a governance system for the care of a 'deteriorating patient' and as a support network for patients that have been discharged from critical care. Patient early warning systems and delivery of sepsis bundles frequently come under the remit of critical care outreach. These nurses will usually have another layer of training and development centred on resuscitation, assessment of deteriorating patients, physical examination and history taking. Decision making around end of life and 'do not attempt resuscitation' falls under the umbrella of the critical care outreach nurse. Early warning systems and deteriorating patient processes repeatedly alert frail, end-stage disease and dying patients to the attention of critical care outreach. Admission prevention by optimising early resuscitation as well as enabling early 'do not resuscitate' and end of life discussions is a key role. In circumstances where critical care admission is delayed, a critical care outreach nurse can deliver care wherever the patient is located until a bed can be accessed.

9

Speech and language therapists

ASFA BASHIR, NICOLA PARGETER
AND LUCY WOOD

Speech and Language Therapists are integral to the critical care multi-disciplinary team (MDT) by offering specialist knowledge and skills in the assessment and management of communication and swallowing difficulties. Such difficulties can arise due to the nature of underlying medical conditions or secondary to the use of technologies for prolonging and supporting life. These difficulties can be both short term and long term and require timely and appropriate intervention in order to aid the patient's recovery and rehabilitation.

'Through their detailed knowledge of communication and swallowing, Speech and Language Therapists have a vital role in optimising care, experience and outcome of patients on critical care' (Royal College of Speech and Language Therapists, 2014).

COMMUNICATION DIFFICULTIES

Communication difficulties can have an impact on patient care in a critical care setting through the following:

- Lack of involvement in their own care and decision making
- Frustration in being unable to effectively communicate their needs

- Impact on individuals' psycho-social well-being (Batty, 2009)
- Increased length of stay in ICU due to inability to participate in goal setting, clinical treatment and end of life decisions (Dowdy et al., 1998)

Speech and Language Therapists can facilitate in the management of communication difficulties through the following:

- Prompt assessment and identification of any underlying communication difficulties. This may include early identification of any possible laryngeal injuries that may warrant further referral for a clinical assessment of the upper airway (e.g. ENT assessment).
- Specialist advice/treatment/strategies to maximise or facilitate the communication ability for the individual alongside useful strategies that could be adopted by family/members of the MDT to aid this.
- Use of alternative communication aids, speaking valves, involvement in decisions about adjustment of ventilator modes to aid expressive output (Sutt et al., 2015).
- Capacity assessment to identify comprehension/language/cognitive impairments that may hinder an individual's ability to engage in this discussion.

SWALLOWING DIFFICULTIES

The prevalence of swallowing difficulties in the critical care population is not uncommon and can arise as a result of muscle weakness, prolonged intubation and procedures such as tracheostomy. Recent literature has identified a high percentage range (50%–70%) of aspiration risk in this population with an increased risk of silent aspiration (i.e. no overt signs of airway compromise being displayed) (Hafner et al., 2008). As a result of this, early identification and management of any underlying dysphagia is essential in preventing complications that could be life threatening (e.g. aspiration pneumonia).

Speech and Language Therapists play a vital role in timely assessment and management of dysphagia and can help minimise complications that could arise as a result of this. This can be provided by the following:

- Specialist assessment and evaluation of the swallow function including the use of objective assessments such as fibre-optic endoscopic evaluation of swallowing (FEES) or videofluoroscopy as required

- Facilitating the weaning process in tracheostomy patients through early identification of secretion management and suitability for cuff deflation trials (Warnecke, 2013)
- Specialist advice on treatment and management of any identified dysphagia (i.e. diet/fluid modification, direct therapy interventions to rehabilitate the swallow and/or postural advice to optimise swallow function)

Communication and swallowing difficulties can cause significant levels of distress in the critical care population and therefore require appropriate access to a suitably qualified Speech and Language Therapist as part of the multi-disciplinary team to minimise this impact.

FURTHER READING

Batty, Sally. "Communication, Swallowing and Feeding in the Intensive Care Unit Patient." *Nursing in Critical* 14, no. 4 (June 2009): 175–179.

Dowdy, Melvin D., Charles Robertson, and John A. Bander. "A Study of Proactive Ethics Consultation for Critically and Terminally Ill Patients with Extended Lengths Of Stay." *Critical Care Medicine* 26, no. 2 (February 1998): 252–259.

Hafner, Gert, Andreas Neuhuber, Sylvia Hirtenfelder, Brigitte Schmedler, and Hans Edmund Eckel. "Fiberoptic Endoscopic Evaluation of Swallowing in Intensive Care Unit Patients." *European Archives of Oto-rhino-laryngology* 265, no. 4 (April 2008): 441–446.

Royal College of Speech and Language Therapists. *Speech and Language Therapy in Adult* Critical *Care. RCSLT Position Paper 2014.* London: Royal College of Speech and Language Therapists, 2014.

Sutt, Anna-Liisa, Petrea Cornwell, Daniel Mullany, Toni Kinneally, and John F. Fraser. "The Use of Tracheostomy Speaking Valves in Mechanically Ventilated Patients Results in Improved Communication and Does Not Prolong Ventilation Time in Cardiothoracic Intensive Care Unit Patients." *Journal of Critical Care* 30, no. 3 (June 2015): 491–494.

Warnecke, Tobias, Sonja Suntrup, Inga K. Teismann, Christina Hamacher, Stephan Oelenberg, and Rainer Dziewas. "Standardized Endoscopic Swallowing Evaluation for Tracheostomy Decannulation in Critically Ill Neurologic Patients." *Critical Care Medicine* 41, no. 7 (July 2013): 1728–1732.

10

The critical care physiotherapist

SARAH BUNTING

Physiotherapy is an integral component of the multidisciplinary management of patients in intensive care units (ICUs); however, the role and treatment methods vary between hospitals due to staffing levels, local approaches and experience. Some of these variations are being addressed following the publication of the NHS England service specification (D16) and GPICS standards.

Survival rate following admission to ICU is increasing due to advances in medical care but this is also increasing the number of patients with long-term physical impairments. Assessment encompasses the respiratory, musculoskeletal, cardiovascular and neurological needs of the patient. Physiotherapists are uniquely qualified with skills and expertise to work with the assessment and management of respiratory complications, physical deconditioning, and neuromuscular and musculoskeletal conditions.

The traditional role of the physiotherapist was the respiratory management of both intubated and spontaneously breathing patients; however, the long-standing physical impairments affecting the survivors of ICU has led to a greater accent on exercise rehabilitation including early mobilisation.

RESPIRATORY TREATMENT

'Eighteen hours of mechanical ventilation leads to structural and functional changes in the diaphragm musculature' (Schepens et al., 2015).

One part of the role of the physiotherapist is to prevent/treat respiratory infections and promote lung function.

Treatments are aimed at

- Secretion removal
- Improved lung compliance/function
- Alveolar recruitment

Techniques for optimisation of cardiopulmonary function include

- Manual hyperinflation (MHI)
- Suction
- Manual techniques: chest shaking and vibration, chest wall compression, positioning
- Active cycle of breathing technique (ACBT)
- Intermittent positive-pressure breathing (IPPB)
- Cough Assist (MI:E)
- Mobilisation/rehabilitation

REHABILITATION

'If immobility is pathology then movement is medicine' (Ridgeway, 2014).

There are multiple challenges to mobility in the ICU setting, including a patient's acuity, the use of sedation, communication with other caregivers and time limitations; however, early rehabilitation is key to improving patients' muscle strength and overall physical function, both during and after their acute illness. Rehabilitation commences whilst the patient is sedated with passive movements to minimise joint stiffness and soft tissue contractures, advancing to active exercises as soon as the patient is able to participate. Every day on bed rest reduces muscle mass by one to three per cent, and this may be higher in the first two weeks of ICU admission. Each patient should receive an individualised, structured rehabilitation programme with a weekly review of his or her goals and outcome measures.

WHAT WE NEED FROM YOU

- Discuss a weaning plan for the patient.
- Discuss whether the patient is ready for extubation/decannulation.
- Is the patient stable for rehabilitation?
- Are you planning any procedures on the patient that requires them to be in bed – so we know when we can sit the patient out?

FURTHER READING

The Faculty of Intensive Care Medicine/The Intensive Care Society. *Guidelines for the Provision of Intensive Care Services*. London: The Faculty of Intensive Care Medicine, 2013. www.ficm.ac.uk /standards-and-guidelines/gpics.

National Institute for Health and Clinical Excellence. *Rehabilitation after Critical Illness, CG83*. London: National Institute for Health and Clinical Excellence, 2009. www.nice.org.uk/CG83.

NHS England Commissioning. "D16 Adult Critical Care." www.england.nhs.uk /commissioning/spec-services/npc-crg/group-d/d05/.

Ridgeway, Kyle. "Physical Therapists in the ICU: ACTION for #ICUrehab# AcutePT." *PT Think Tank* (2 November 2014). https://ptthinktank.com /2014/11/02/physical-therapists-in-the-icu-action-for-icurehab-acutept/.

Schepens, Tom, Walter Verbrugghe, Karolien Dams, Bob Corthouts, Paul M. Parizel and Philippe G. Jorens. "The Course of Diaphragm Atrophy in Ventilated Patients Assessed with Ultrasound: A Longitudinal Cohort Study." *Critical Care* 19 (December 2015): 422. https://ccforum .biomedcentral.com/articles/10.1186/s13054-015-1141-0 (accessed 10 Nov 2017).

11

Advanced critical care practitioners (ACCP)

GAVIN DENTON

BACKGROUND

Advanced nurse practitioner (ANP) roles have been evolving in the United Kingdom for over 20 years. They have developed in a multitude of areas in both primary and secondary care sectors. In many ways, this process was accelerated when non-medical prescribing was introduced to nursing in the 1990s. Frequently, advanced nurse practitioner roles were filled by lone mavericks who forged their particular roles on an individual basis. Over the years, medical specialties began to consider these roles on a more systematic level. The implementation of the European Union working time directive (WTD) provided a second stimulus to the burgeoning role of ANPs. Concerns about the impact of the WTD on the medical workforce population and the ability to meet future health care demands lead to individual trusts and services considering diversifying their medical workforce in an effort to secure the ability to meet the demands placed on services. In recognition of these concerns, the Department of Health produced a competency framework for advanced nurse practitioners working in critical care (Department of Health, 2008). This framework was designed to unify the competence of nurses working in advanced roles in critical care.

RECOGNITION BY THE FACULTY OF INTENSIVE CARE MEDICINE

In 2015, the Faculty of Intensive Care Medicine (FICM) produced its own competency framework whereby on completion the individual would be registered with FICM as an advanced critical care practitioner, or ACCP for short (FICM, 2015). In addition to this, FICM has also produced a continuing professional development and appraisal framework (FICM, 2015). ACCPs who were established in their roles prior to the FICM pathway can register as associates of FICM after a portfolio submission process. Registration with FICM is not mandatory; however, it is envisioned that this process will provide a universal standard of training and practice, while also ensuring that practitioners are actually portable across the NHS and not just within the institutions that trained them.

WHAT ARE THE TYPICAL BACKGROUNDS OF ACCPs?

ACCPs are typically from a nursing background; however, this is not universal and there are trainees with backgrounds in para-medicine and physiotherapy. The typical ACCP is an experienced nurse from the critical care environment; many will have worked at charge nurse level for some years in critical care. Prior to training, most nurses will have already completed a diploma, often at degree level in critical care nursing. Training of ACCPs is at the master's level, and involves non-medical prescribing, training in examination and history taking, diagnostics and investigations, resuscitation and transfer of the critically ill. Training should be at least two years and in a fully supernumerary capacity. Medical oversight should be with a consultant in critical care and include continuous mentoring and supervision.

CURRENT ROLES OF THE CRITICAL CARE PRACTITIONERS WITHIN CRITICAL CARE SERVICES

ACCPs are not a replacement but a complement to the traditional medical roles within the critical care team. The role encompasses much of the care delivered by both junior and middle grade doctors within a critical care service. Participation in multidisciplinary ward rounds, all aspects of pre-scribing within critical care, referring and liaising between clinical teams, ordering diagnostics and investigations are typical routine roles of ACCPs. Most procedures typical to critical care can be carried out by ACCPs with the exception of independent provision of anaesthesia. These procedures include invasive vascular access, intercostal drain insertions, transfer of critically ill ventilated patients and intubation (not independently). ACCPs will often form part of on-call resuscitation teams, providing either leadership or air-way management, and will often provide inter-hospital transfer and retrieval services. In some centres, critical care outreach provision is also part of the wider role of ACCPs. Qualified ACCPs are also a significant learning and supervision resource for junior doctors rotating through the critical care ser-vices, whether that is support, teaching or supervision of procedures.

ADDITIONAL ADVANTAGES OF ACCPs

The medical workforce of any critical care service is extremely transient, with consultants being the only consistent element to the medical team. This pres-ents particular problems in maintaining consistency, especially in compli-ance to unit specific policies and procedures. The addition of ACCPs to the critical care medical workforce ameliorates some of these problems especially during out-of-hours working.

FURTHER READING

The Faculty of Intensive Care Medicine. *Advanced Critical Care Practitioners: CPD and Appraisal Pathway*. London: The Faculty of Intensive Care Medicine, 2016. https://www.ficm.ac.uk/sites/default/files/accp_cpd_appraisal _pathway_-_version_1_-_july_2016.pdf (accessed 10 October 2016).

The Faculty of Intensive Care Medicine. *Curriculum for Training Advanced Critical Care Practitioners*. London: The Faculty of Intensive Care Medicine, 2015. https://www.ficm.ac.uk/sites/default/files/ACCP%20 Curriculum%20v1.0%20(2015)%20COMPLETE_0.pdf (accessed 10 October 2016).

The Faculty of Intensive Care Medicine. Department of Health. *The National Education and Competence Framework for Advanced Critical Care Practitioners. A Discussion Document*. London: The Faculty of Intensive Care Medicine, 2008.

The critical care pharmacist

ADEYEMI OYEDELE

Clinical pharmacy (pharmacists and technicians) in critical care has evolved over the past three decades to become an integral part of the multidisciplinary critical care team (Intensive Care Society and The Faculty of Intensive Care Medicine, 2016; Shulman et al., 2015). It is well established in the care of the critically ill patient that a critical care pharmacist plays an important role in improving the safe and effective use of medicines (Bourne et al., 2016). This is recognised in the guidelines for the provision of intensive care services (GPICS) that states that there must be a critical care pharmacist for every critical care unit who also contributes to the daily consultant-led ward round (Intensive Care Society and The Faculty of Intensive Care Medicine, 2016).

In the critically ill patient, frequent formulation and dose changes of medicines are required due to various patient-related factors and the specialty of critical care (Shulman, 2015; Bourne et al., 2016). They are exposed to a great amount of enteral and parenteral medicines, on complex pharmaceutical regimens, are prone to drug–drug and drug–food interactions, have acute changes in organ function and may need extracorporeal modalities such as renal replacement therapy (Bourne et al., 2016). This necessitates the need for a pharmacist to improve medicines-related patient outcomes and reduce adverse events. A pharmacist's intervention in critical care is associated with prevention and detection of medication errors and optimisation of medication therapy.

Unintentional medication omission is a potential for harm and a source of medication error on admission to a hospital (Barrett et al., 2012). An effective strategy to prevent this is medicines reconciliation, which is the process of obtaining and communicating 'the most accurate list of a patient's current medicines (including drug name, dosage, frequency and route), comparing them to the current list in use and recognising and document-ing any changes and discrepancies' (National Institute for Health and Care Excellence, 2015). Although the acute medical problem with which a patient presents to critical care is the primary focus of care, discrepancies relating to omission of medication used to control long-term health conditions should be reviewed and resolved promptly by the doctors before a patient is dis-charged from critical care.

Critical care pharmacists optimise the impact of medicines prescribed during daily individual patient medication review and attendance on ward rounds. This ensures the best possible outcome for patients (Shulman et al., 2015; National Institute for Health and Care Excellence, 2015). Medicines optimisation comprise proactive intervention such as a critical care phar-macist initiated recommendation, adjustment or addition to enhance the effectiveness and safety of pharmacotherapy (Shulman et al., 2015). Other common interventions include therapeutic drug monitoring, supra- or sub-therapeutic drug doses, drug interactions, issues of intravenous compatibil-ity, enteral feeding tube administration, antimicrobial stewardship, adverse drug reaction and nonconformity to formulary/guidelines (Shulman et al., 2015; Richter et al., 2016).

Additional roles of the critical care pharmacist include drug-use evalua-tion, provision of in-service education for nurses and doctors and nutrition team participation (Richter et al., 2016). The GPICS encourage critical care pharmacists to become independent prescribers. This allows them to pre-scribe within their level of experience and sphere of competence (Intensive Care Society and The Faculty of Intensive Care Medicine, 2016; Shulman et al., 2015; Bourne et al., 2016).

FURTHER READING

Barrett, Nicholas A., Andrew Jones, Craig Whiteley, Sarah Yassin, and Catherine A. McKenzie. "Management of Long-Term Hypothyroidism: A Potential Marker of Quality of Medicines Reconciliation in the Intensive Care Unit." *International Journal of Pharmacy Practice* 20, no. 5 (May 2012): 303–306.

Bourne, Richard S., Paul Whiting, Lisa S. Brown, and Mark Borthwick. "Pharmacist Independent Prescribing in Critical Care: Results of a National Questionnaire to Establish the 2014 UK Position." *International Journal of Pharmacy Practice* 24, no. 2 (September 2015): 104–113.

The Intensive Care Society and The Faculty of Intensive Care Medicine. *Guidelines for the Provision of Intensive Care Services*. Edition 1.1. London: The Faculty of Intensive Care Medicine, 2016.

National Institute for Health and Care Excellence. *Medicines Optimisation: The Safe and Effective Use of Medicines to Enable the Best Possible Outcomes*. NICE Guideline (NG5). London: NICE; 2015.

Richter, Anja, Ian Bates, Meera Thacker, Yogini Jani, Bryan O'Farrell, Caroline Edwards, Helen Taylor, and Rob Shulman. "Impact of the Introduction of a Specialist Critical Care Pharmacist on the Level of Pharmaceutical Care Provided to the Critical Care Unit." *International Journal of Pharmacy Practice* 24, no. 4 (August 2016): 253–261.

Shulman, Rob, Catherine A. McKenzie, June Landa, Richard S. Bourne, Andrew Jones, Mark Borthwick, Mark Tomlin, Yogini H. Jani, David West, and Ian Bates, for the PROTECTED-UK Group. "Pharmacist's Review and Outcomes: Treatment-Enhancing Contributions Tallied, Evaluated, and Documented (PROTECTED-UK)." *Journal of Critical Care* 30, no. 4 (August 2015): 808–813.

PART ③

INITIAL ASSESSMENT
The first hour

13

Assessing ICU referrals on the ward

CATRIONA FRANKLING AND JOYCE YEUNG

'Please could you come and see Mr Smith on ward 10? I think he needs to go to intensive care. He's too sick to stay on our ward!'

ICU referrals on the ward can be anything, from a young patient with sepsis, to an elderly patient with an exacerbation of chronic obstructive pulmonary disease (COPD). However, the assessment for any of these patients remains the same, and is best approached systematically to ensure a thorough assessment. Following your assessment, an appropriate management plan can be made and communicated to the ward staff.

If possible, gather as much information as you can before visiting the ward, including basic information such as age, name and hospital number (so that you can view imaging or pathology results) as well as current observations. Ideally, any referrals via telephone should follow a structured approach such as SBAR (situation, background, assessment and recommendation) from the referring health professional so that workload can be prioritised. Whilst ICU can be a busy job, it is always recommended that you personally see and assess all patients that are referred.

USING A SYSTEMATIC APPROACH TO ASSESS REFERRALS

The simplest method for assessment is to follow 'ABCDE'. This ensures that nothing is missed, and may be more appropriate in emergency referrals to ensure that any urgent issues, such as airway compromise, are dealt with first. An alternative approach involves the conventional medical assessment of presenting complaint, history of presenting complaint, past medical history, etc. However, many ICU referrals from the ward are more urgent, lending themselves to the 'ABC' approach.

AIRWAY

Listen for any sounds that suggest an obstructed airway, such as snoring. Remember that a completely occluded airway will be silent. Look at the chest movement – obstruction can lead to paradoxical 'see-saw' chest and abdominal movement. Airway obstruction is an emergency so call for help straight away. An obstructed airway can often be relieved with simple airway manoeuvres, such as head tilt and chin lift, as described in basic life support guidelines. Expert help will be needed for more advanced airway management.

BREATHING

Introduce yourself to the patient and ask them some open-ended questions about their current medical problems. This will give you the patient's history, and will demonstrate whether they can complete long or short sentences, or are too breathless to speak for long. What is their respiratory rate and oxygen saturations? Is the patient on oxygen? And if so, do they keep it on? Examine their respiratory system. Make note of any respiratory medications and any recent arterial blood gas results. Look at any recent chest x-rays. It is appropriate to address any issues as you find them, for example if the patient is hypoxic, then start oxygen therapy at 15 L/min via a non-rebreathe mask, then titrate down based on the pulse oximetry. Oxygen saturations of 94%–98% are appropriate in acute respiratory failure. If the patient is at risk of type 2 respiratory failure, then aim for oxygen saturations of 88%–92%.

CIRCULATION

Find out the patient's heart rate and blood pressure. Listen to the heart sounds. Is the patient peripherally warm and what is the capillary refill time? What is the urine output and fluid balance? If the examination reveals that the patient is under-filled, administer a fluid challenge. Stay with the patient to assess the results of your fluid challenge – any changes to heart rate or blood pressure may only be transient if they remain under-filled. If the examination suggests heart failure (bi-basal crackles on chest auscultation, raised JVP or third heart sound), then stop or decrease intravenous fluid infusions. If there is chest pain and acute coronary syndrome (ACS) is suspected, then treat for ACS. Remember to look at any recent electrocardiograms (ECGs), and ask for a new ECG recording if there is any suspicion of ACS or arrhythmias.

DISABILITY

Assess the patient's level of consciousness. This can initially be assessed rapidly using AVPU (Alert, responds to Vocal stimuli, responds to Painful stimuli, Unresponsive). The Glasgow Coma Scale can also be used to assess their conscious level. Causes for depressed conscious level can include hypoxia, hypercapnia, hypotension (leading to decreased cerebral perfusion), sedatives and hypoglycaemia. Check the patient's drug chart for medications such as morphine that can reduce conscious level. Consider administering naloxone if appropriate. Check the blood glucose rapidly using finger-prick bedside testing. Hypoglycaemia can be treated with 50 mL of 10% glucose intravenously. Is the patient orientated to time and place or have they developed new onset confusion? Acute confusion and changes in conscious level can both signify deterioration in patients. Depressed conscious level can lead to airway compromise, so consider seeking expert help from an anaesthetist if the airway is not protected. Nurse in the lateral position until the airway is protected.

EXPOSURE

Fully examine the patient whilst respecting their dignity and minimising heat loss. Check the patient's temperature. Remember that severe sepsis can lead to hypothermia as well as pyrexia. Look for other clues on exposure, such as sacral pressure sores, which could be a source of infection and hints at the patient's functional status.

ADDITIONAL INFORMATION

Speak to the patient, relatives and ward staff to find out the patient's clinical history. Read the medical notes; if this is long and time is limited, focus on recent entries, the initial clerking for the current admission, clinic letters (which help establish the severity of any chronic illnesses and may outline discussed treatment limitations) and any previous ICU admissions. Speak to the patient and their family about their treatment and prognosis. This may include a discussion about the patient's wishes about resuscitation, and whether they want to have interventions such as intubation. It is also important to explore the patient's and family's expectations to ensure both the patient and their relatives understand what can realistically be achieved by medical intervention. If a 'do not attempt resuscitation' (DNAR) order is part of your management plan, this must be discussed with the patient. If the patient lacks capacity to understand the DNAR decision, then it must be discussed with the family instead.

MAKING A PLAN

To make a plan it may be easier to think in terms of immediate plans for the ward and the need for ICU.

IMMEDIATE PLAN FOR THE WARD

This may include oxygen therapy, intravenous fluids, antibiotics, or repeating investigations such as arterial blood gases. Document your findings, diagnoses and management plan clearly in the notes. It is also important to tell the ward staff your findings and plans, as they may not check the notes straight away, especially if you want the ward staff to carry out part of your management plan! Make it clear what will happen next – for example, will the critical care outreach team come and review the patient in two hours, or will the patient be transferred to ICU immediately or when a bed becomes available? Sometimes, the ward team may not agree with your management plan. If this happens, explain your reasoning for your current plan, and listen to why they do not agree with it. You may find that they have a valid argument and you can change your plan accordingly. If you are still not in agreement, discuss it with the consultant in charge of ICU. Some patients can be complex and deciding on a management plan may not be easy. Seek help and support from your seniors if you are unsure.

THE NEED FOR ICU

Discuss your assessment and findings with the ICU consultant. Try to rationalise whether the patient needs ICU treatment and, if so, what treatments will be required. Use the SBAR method for communicating your findings. Typically there will be one of three options for the patient:

- The patient does not require ICU and can be managed on the ward. They may still have the potential to deteriorate and require ICU care. A plan should be made for a member of the ICU team to review the patient. The ward should be instructed to call ICU if the patient deteriorates.
- The patient requires ICU care and can no longer be managed on the ward. Find out from the nurse in charge of ICU if there is a bed available immediately or if there will be a delay. Consider who will be needed to transfer the patient – do you need an anaesthetist or can they be transferred safely without someone with advanced airway skills? Make sure you have all the necessary equipment for transfer. If there will be a delay, discuss with the ICU consultant what care the patient needs in the interim. This may involve review from the critical care outreach team.
- The patient is not a suitable candidate for ICU. This may be because of an irreversible disease process, or it may be that the patient does not wish to have ICU care. These can be tricky situations. There are no definitive rules so discuss all cases with the ICU consultant. The ICU consultant will want to know the ward team's prognosis for the patient, the patient's functional status and the patient's and family's expectations and wishes. If the patient refuses ICU care, it is important to find out why. If they do not want to be intubated, but would accept inotropic support or

non-invasive ventilation, then they may still be suitable for ICU but with limitations on treatment. Clearly document the reasons for limitations on treatment and ensure any specific paperwork is completed fully.

KEY LEARNING POINTS

- Clear communication is vital, including with the referring health professional, the ward team, the patient and their family, and the ICU consultant.
- A systematic approach to assessment using ABCDE ensures that nothing is missed.
- Discuss the management plan with the ICU consultant. Document the plan clearly in your notes and tell the ward team your plan.

FURTHER READING

Makings, Ellen. "HDU and ICU care." In Catherine Spoors and Kevin Kiff (eds.), *Training in Anaesthesia: The Essential Curriculum*, 528–529. Oxford: Oxford University Press, 2015.

Resuscitation Council (UK). "Non-Technical Skills in Resuscitation." In *Advanced Life Support, Seventh Edition*, 712. London: Resuscitation Council, 2016a.

Resuscitation Council (UK). "Recognising Deterioration and Preventing Cardiorespiratory Arrest." In *Advanced Life Support, Seventh Edition*, 13–22. London: Resuscitation Council, 2016b.

14

Assessment and management of major trauma patients

IAN TYRELL-MARSH AND EDWARD DENISON-DAVIES

It is late and you are working in your local Major Trauma Centre (MTC). You are called to the Emergency Department (ED) as part of the trauma team. In ED, the staff tells you that a 25-year-old man has been hit by a car; he has suspected head and chest injuries. When the prehospital team arrives, you are presented with a patient on a scoop stretcher with cervical collar, blocks and a pelvic splint applied. He has obvious bruising around the face. His airway is partially obstructed, his respiratory rate is 28, and saturations are 99% on 15L via a non-rebreathe mask (NRB). He has marked crepitus on palpation of the right-hand side of his chest and a good radial pulse. The general surgeon confirms his abdomen is soft and non-tender. The orthopaedic surgeon states he appears to have no femoral or humeral injuries. You confirm his GCS as being E2, V2, M4. His pupils are equal and reactive to light.

What do you do next?

INTRODUCTION

Major trauma is responsible for over 3000 deaths per year and it remains the leading cause of death in people under the age of 40 in the UK. The centralisation of Major Trauma services into an MTC (Major Trauma Centre)/TU (Trauma Unit) hub and spoke model has meant that although patients travel a little further, their access to advanced services such as interventional radiology, neurosurgical facilities, appropriate intensive care, physiotherapy and rehabilitation services is much improved. A Trauma Audit and Research Network (TARN) audit in 2014 claimed this redesign has saved over 600 lives per year[1].

This chapter aims to give you an understanding of the initial C (catastrophic haemorrhage), ABC assessment of the trauma patient as well as some of the management strategies that are used.

THE EMERGENCY DEPARTMENT

The purpose of the trauma call alert is to assemble a multi-disciplinary team in good time to ensure rapid assessment of a trauma patient. You can expect an ED senior doctor (often team leader), anaesthetist/intensivist, general surgeon and orthopaedic doctor as a minimum along with at least two ED nurses. Grades of doctor vary significantly, and as you would expect in the MTCs, those present are likely to be more senior (registrar or consultant level). Specific specialties are unlikely to be available in all hospitals.

In the time before the patient arrives, team introductions are essential, so people have an idea of who everyone is and their skill set. Some centres have colour-coded stickers to be worn that help identify specialties. Try to identify where specific equipment is kept in case you need it emergently; this includes drugs. Some places will provide a 'grab box' of the likely drugs required; however, the team may also need access to ED stock for fridge items or less commonly used medications.

PATIENT ARRIVAL

Depending on the severity of injury, seniority and confidence of the treating pre-hospital team, patients will arrive with differing levels of treatment. Most will arrive on a scoop stretcher; this is superior to a spinal board with a lesser degree of pressure sore formation and the ability to 'split' the scoop top and bottom to separate it into two bladed sides. This allows for minimal handling of the patient to get them onto the board, thus reducing the risk of clot dis-lodgement during handling.

CERVICAL SPINE CONTROL

Most patients regardless of mechanism or symptoms will have had a cervical collar, head blocks and tape applied. Over the next five years we may see a sharp decline in the use of cervical collars and currently many practitioners actively avoid placing one due to problems with pressure sores, impedance of airway management and the poor evidence base.

If the patient is combative, they are likely to require intubation as they will almost certainly require a CT scan. Up until anaesthesia, minimal restraint should be used and interventions that may cause distress or discomfort avoided, as this will cause further rises in intracranial pressure and risks injury to both staff and patient. Once anaesthetized, blocks and tape should then be applied. A detailed neurological exam should be conducted prior to anaesthesia. Although progression of symptoms during resuscitation and intubation is unusual, swelling around the spinal cord can produce a rising neurological level.

PRIMARY SURVEY

The objective of the primary survey is to diagnose life-threatening airway, breathing or circulation problems, as there are conditions that are important to pick up prior to a trauma CT, which may require the patient to bypass CT to go for interventional radiology (IR) or theatre first.

Teams operate in different ways with some teams dividing the responsibility of the primary survey between several clinicians. It is the authors' opinion that the survey is best done by a single clinician as this

- Ensures continuity, meaning a single system is followed and features are less likely to be missed
- Requires fewer bodies around the patient
- Enables clear communication from the clinician to the scribe/trauma team leader

Ideally the findings of the survey should be communicated to the whole team so everyone is aware of their presence and significance. It is also helpful if a summary is broadcast after the survey is complete to focus the team on the task at hand.

CATASTROPHIC HAEMORRHAGE

Catastrophic haemorrhage requiring immediate treatment is relatively rare within civilian practice in the UK. Examples may include some arterial or vena caval vascular injuries, significant pelvic injuries or large intra-abdominal solid organ injuries such as extensive splenic or liver lacerations. The majority of these patients, if bleeding is non-compressible and rapid, will exsanguinate prior to arrival in hospital and their presenting complaint is likely to be traumatic cardiac arrest.

AIRWAY

Assessment of the airway should take no longer than 30 seconds. Simply asking the patient their name will provide cues that the airway is clear if there is a change of quality in their voice (in the case of burns or laryngeal trauma) or if there is the presence of shortness of breath or respiratory embarrassment.

If airway compromise is present, it must be treated aggressively and without delay. Have a low threshold for the use of basic airway adjuncts such as Guedel and nasopharyngeal (NP) airways if the patient's GCS will allow. The gold standard is two NP airways and a Guedel airway to maximise airway patency with a two-person technique utilising an assistant to squeeze the bag until a formal airway can be established. A base-of-skull fracture is not a contraindication for an NP airway, and if a patient has a head injury significant enough to cause a fracture, their chance of intracranial haematoma is in the region of 20%; the risk benefit for avoidance of hypoxia is in favour of insertion of an airway. *The goal is always to oxygenate the patient adequately* in preparation for definitive airway management (rapid sequence intubation).

BREATHING

Good inspection of the chest wall for deformities and bruising combined with the mechanism of injury can help focus the chest examination; look for seatbelt marks in particular. The patient's respiratory rate, depth and effort as well as oxygen requirements should be noted.

The chest should be palpated, systematically examining each rib. Check for tenderness, crepitus and surgical emphysema to indicate rib fractures and potential underlying pneumothorax or lung contusion. Rib fractures can lead to damage to underlying organs (lung/liver/spleen).

Auscultation of the chest can reveal decreased breath sounds indicative of a pneumothorax or haemothorax. A small pneumothorax can present with unilateral wheeze only. If a pneumothorax is suspected, drainage may be required via an intercostal drain. Decompression for a tension pneumothorax is ideally done in the same manner though some clinicians may initially use a cannula in the mid-clavicular line, second intercostal space. If a cannula is placed, it should be converted to an intercostal drain as soon as possible.

CIRCULATION

The aim of the circulatory assessment is to assess whether the patient requires resuscitation before heading to the CT scanner, or if they are so unstable they require direct transfer to interventional radiology or theatre.

Begin by palpating the radial/brachial/central pulse; this will give a guide as to an approximate blood pressure (90/70/60 mmHg). Check capillary refill and temperature and palpate the abdomen for tenderness or rigidity. Have a high index of suspicion for retroperitoneal bleeding, which has few if any signs but can lead to significant shock.

If a pelvic binder is in situ, leave it in place; an assessment can be made around the device. Check for symmetry across the pelvis. Do not 'spring' the pelvis as this dislodges the clot. Palpate the pubic symphysis for tenderness and inspect the external genitalia, perineum and anus for the presence of blood (indicative of a pelvic fracture).

Significant blood can be lost into long bone compartments and the limbs should be examined for deformity, tenderness or crepitus. If a displaced fracture is identified, splintage may be required to limit ongoing blood loss.

RAPID SEQUENCE INTUBATION IN THE EMERGENCY DEPARTMENT

Rapid Sequence Intubation (RSI) describes the process by which the airway is secured by placement of an endotracheal tube in the shortest possible time from induction of anaesthesia, to minimise risk of regurgitation and aspiration. It is used in patients that have been unable to be starved.

The process of RSI is inherently risky as loss of the airway in a paralysed patient can rapidly lead to desaturation and death, and many of the drugs used cause cardiovascular instability. It does, however, allow oxygenation and ventilation of the patient and facilitates other invasive procedures that the patient may require.

Given the complexity and inherent risk involved around intubation, many hospitals are moving towards the use of a pre-intubation checklist to improve safety. An example, the B@EASE checklist, is shown in Figure 14.1. Regardless of which checklist is in use at your hospital, be familiar with it and expect to use it during any airway procedure (trauma or otherwise) in the emergency department, intensive care or remote site.

The drugs used in theatre can also be used for emergency anaesthesia, although the vasodilatory effects of many of the agents are undesirable especially in the hypovolaemic patient. A rapid acting muscle relaxant is also required; either suxamethonium or a higher dose of rocuronium is an acceptable choice. Many clinicians are gaining experience with the use of ketamine in major trauma. Ketamine's cardiovascular profile is more forgiving than other induction agents. It is also an excellent analgesic and can be used in smaller doses (0.1–0.5 mg/kg) to facilitate manipulation of angulated fractures or for unpleasant invasive procedures. Commonly used emergency intubating drug doses are shown in Figure 14.2.

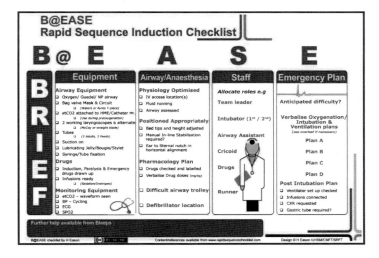

Figure 14.1 The B@EASE checklist.

Fentanyl	1–3 mcg/kg
Ketamine	1–2 mg/kg
Rocuronium	1 mg/kg
Thiopentone	3–7 mg/kg
Suxamethonium	1–2 mg/kg

Figure 14.2 Intubation drug doses.

WHERE DO THEY GO NEXT?

There are essentially two options for the major trauma patient from the resus room. Most patients will now go to the CT scanner for definitive imaging and identification of their overall injury load. When a definitive list has been collated, specialist teams can be asked for their input to organise management of the specific injuries. Some of these patients will go direct to theatre; others will go to the major trauma ward or critical care.

For those patients that are too unstable to go to the CT scanner, ongoing resuscitation will be required in tandem with an effort to arrest the cause of bleeding. The two most frequently used options are either direct to theatre for damage control surgery or to the interventional radiology suite for embolisation of arterial bleeding.

CASE REVIEW

Think back to the case at the beginning of the chapter. Below is one possible management plan.

This patient has a significant mechanism of injury, combined with a reduced GCS and signs of a right-sided pneumothorax. He is cardiovascularly stable and hence the most likely hospital pathway is via the CT scanner. To facilitate this he will require an anaesthetic to protect his airway and neuroprotective ventilation for his suspected significant head injury.

He is highly likely to have a right-sided pneumothorax, which may well get worse with positive pressure ventilation after intubation. A low threshold for decompression and intercostal drain insertion is sensible. As the patient is cardiovascularly stable, urgent decompression pre-intubation is not required.

KEY LEARNING POINTS

- Effective, timely management of the poly-trauma patient requires a multi-disciplinary approach with robust decision making and good team leadership.
- The primary survey is essential to rule out any immediately life-threatening injuries.
- Most patients will have a whole body CT scan from head to pelvis to help in the identification of injury load and planning of further management.
- Some patients may be too unstable for CT and will need to go directly to interventional radiology or theatre for life-saving interventions.

FURTHER READING

American College of Surgeons. Advanced Trauma Life Support (ATLS®) Program. Chicago: American College of Surgeons, 2017. www.facs.org /quality-programs/trauma/atls.

European Resuscitation Council (ERC), European Society of Anaesthesiology (ESA), European Society for Trauma and Emergency Surgery (ESTES), and European Society for Emergency Medicine (EuSEM). "European Trauma Course – The Team Approach to Trauma." http://europeantraumacourse.com/.

National Health Service (NHS) England. "News: NHS Saves Lives of Hundreds More Trauma Victims Just Two Years After Changes to Care – Independent Audit." *NHS England* (1 July 2014). www.england .nhs.uk/2014/07/trauma-independent-audit/.

15

Management of the head-injured patient

KUNAL LUND AND THOMAS OWEN

'Would you mind coming and having a quick look at Mrs Smith in resus? She slipped and bumped her head this morning. She was fine initially and just awaiting a CT scan. In the last hour, she's become quite drowsy and dropped her GCS. I'm not happy to take her for a scan by myself'.

Each year approximately 1–1.4 million people attend emergency departments in England and Wales with a head injury. Whilst 95% of these people will have an injury classed as 'minor', around 200,000 people will still require hospital admission, with an estimated 3500 of them requiring an ICU admission. Traumatic brain injury is associated with a very significant morbidity and mortality. It is the commonest cause of death and disability in people aged 1–40, and accounts for 1% of all adult deaths in the UK. Survivors of significant head injuries can often be left with lifelong disability affecting them cognitively, emotionally and physically. The overall impact on a patient can be catastrophic.

This chapter will focus on the initial assessment and management of head injured patients, followed by the main principles of managing these patients on an intensive care unit.

BASIC PRINCIPLES

Brain injury following head trauma may be classified by timing:

- *Primary Injury* – The original insult to the brain that occurred at the time of trauma. There is nothing we can do to alter or influence this.
- *Secondary Injury* – Any subsequent insult to the brain occurring after the initial trauma. This may be caused by a number of factors as listed, and is potentially preventable:
  - Raised intracranial pressure
  - Hypotension
  - Hypoxia
  - Hyper-/hypoglycaemia
  - Hyper-/hypocapnia (High or low $PaCO_2$)
  - Pyrexia

The mainstay of our treatment on intensive care is focused on minimising secondary injury to the brain. As such, it is important that the above factors are considered when assessing any patient. The importance and detailed management of them will be covered below, in the section on specialist critical care management.

Prevention of hypoxia and hypotension are of particular importance as even single, short-lived periods of these have been proven to have detrimental effects on outcomes!

WHAT SHOULD YOU DO IN RESPONSE TO THE NURSE'S QUESTION?

A decrease in GCS in a trauma patient may not necessarily be due to a significant head injury. Certainly, a worsening neurological state may be precipitated by hypovolaemia, hypoxia or pain due to other serious injuries.

Regardless of cause, a decrease in GCS potentially signifies that a patient is critically unwell, and therefore a structured, 'ABC' approach is essential. Remember to call for help early, as these patients can deteriorate quickly without specialist management.

INITIAL ASSESSMENT AND MANAGEMENT (FIRST HOURS)

A: Airway
- Give oxygen at a rate of 15 litres per minute via a non-rebreathe mask with a reservoir bag.
- Immobilise the cervical spine, as there is a high risk of a neck injury.
- Ensure there is a patent, unobstructed airway.
  - An obstructed airway may cause hypoxia/hypercapnia, which can be detrimental to the head-injured patient.
- If the airway cannot be maintained by airway manoeuvres or by an oropharyngeal airway, then they require intubation. Intubation should be performed with manual in-line C-spine immobilisation. (Remember, a nasopharyngeal airway is contraindicated if there is the possibility of a base of skull injury!)

B: Breathing
- Are the rate and depth of breathing adequate? Is the patient hyperventilating? Check oxygen saturations, respiratory rate, and consider arterial blood gases to aid your clinical assessment.
- Consider assisted bag-mask ventilation if breathing is inadequate, and get urgent anaesthetic assistance with consideration for intubation and controlled ventilation.
- Evaluate for any chest injuries (e.g. haemo-/pneumothorax) and manage as appropriate.
- Remember, hypoxia and hypercapnia could be disastrous for a head-injured patient!

C: Circulation
- Assess capillary refill, pulse and blood pressure.
- Resuscitate with intravenous fluids to a normal blood pressure – a single episode of hypotension can have a negative effect on outcomes.

- Is there any evidence of active bleeding from anywhere? If there
  is, consider blood products, aim to control bleeding and contact
  surgeons as a matter of urgency.
- Once the patient is euvolaemic, inotropes or vasopressors may be
  indicated to maintain a normal or even an elevated blood pressure,
  depending on clinical circumstances.

D: Disability

- Determine their Glasgow Coma Scale (GCS; table on page 358).
- If the GCS is 8 or less, then they require intubation and ventilation;
  there is a high risk of aspiration in these patients.
- If the patient is restless or agitated and lacks capacity, they may
  require intubation and ventilation to facilitate imaging or ongoing
  clinical care. (Be very wary about attempting to provide light sedation in these patients as they can deteriorate very quickly and it can
  confuse the clinical picture!)
- Check the size and reaction of the pupils.
- A low GCS and dilated pupil(s) in a head-injured patient is likely
  a sign of significant brain injury and raised intracranial pressure.
  It will almost certainly lead to rapid deterioration and coning if
  left untreated. Consider 20% mannitol (0.25–1 g/kg) or hypertonic
  saline as osmotherapy to 'buy time' until potentially definitive
  treatment. These agents reduce cerebral oedema but are not without
  their risks.
- If there is any evidence of seizure activity, these should be actively
  treated.
- Treat pain with morphine if required.

E: Exposure

- Look for evidence of other injuries, or active bleeding.
- Unless there is a specific indication, active re-warming is not
  required in mild hypothermia.

Imaging

- A CT scan of the head and neck is likely warranted. Consider a
  full trauma CT scan if indicated or if there is evidence of other
  injuries.
- Safely CT scanning a patient with a potentially significant head
  injury requires thorough preparation and stabilisation before

transfer. You should not be pressurised into taking a patient before they are safe.

- If there is an indication to intubate, this should be done prior to transfer. It should be done by someone experienced in performing rapid sequence induction. Transfer to scan should be performed by someone experienced in the management of such patients.
- Remember, even after a patient has been scanned, a further significant drop in GCS (2 or more) may be an indication for repeat imaging!

Transfer to Specialist Centres

- If there is evidence of traumatic brain injury, the patient should be discussed with the regional neurosurgical team.
  - They should be considered for specialist management at a neurosurgical centre even if they do not actively need surgery or critical care.
  - All patients who have evidence of a severe brain injury and who require surgery or critical care should be managed at a specialist centre.
- Transfer should be performed by a practitioner experienced in the management of critically unwell patients. They should ideally also have some experience in the management of trauma and head injuries.

ONGOING CRITICAL CARE MANAGEMENT IN SEVERE TRAUMATIC BRAIN INJURY (HOURS TO DAYS)

The rest of this chapter aims to provide an introduction to the ongoing medical management of the severely brain-injured patient on neuro-critical care. Invariably, these patients will need intubation and ventilation to facilitate their care, and so this should be assumed to be the case for the rest of this chapter.

In addition, whilst the chapter will not expressly cover specific neurosurgical interventions, we must highlight the importance of a close multi-disciplinary team working with the neurosurgical teams, to help identify when surgical intervention is appropriate.

CEREBRAL PERFUSION AND INTRACRANIAL PRESSURE

The principles of critical care management in severe traumatic brain injury are supportive. The majority of the interventions are aimed at maintaining adequate cerebral perfusion to the brain, and thereby minimising secondary injury. This is predominantly done by manipulating factors to try to reduce intracranial pressure (ICP):

$$CPP = MAP - ICP$$

Where CPP is Cerebral Perfusion Pressure and MAP is Mean Arterial Pressure.

Therefore, it can be seen that an adequate CPP can be obtained by maintaining a normal to high MAP but a low ICP. The ideal CPP is approximately 60–70 mmHg, and the ICP is believed to be harmful (regardless of CPP) at a level persistently above 20 mmHg. As such, we should routinely target an ICP of less than 20 mmHg and a MAP of around 70–80 mmHg.

To accurately facilitate this, all traumatic brain injury patients who are admitted to a neuro-critical care should have invasive arterial pressure and ICP monitoring inserted within two hours of arrival. This will allow us to accurately titrate medical therapies to keep the ICP below 20 mmHg.

A stepwise guideline from Level 1 to Level 4 allows us to escalate therapy in a methodical order to try and maintain ICP and CPP targets. If at any point the ICP increases above 20 mmHg for >5 minutes, therapy should be escalated and a consideration taken as to whether repeat scanning or surgery is indicated.

Remember! Level 1 therapy should be started as soon as the patient is intubated, and should not wait for ICP monitoring; it should be started long before they reach a specialist centre!

Level 1 Management:

- Nurse patient's head 30 degrees up in a neutral position. If there is suspicion of spinal injury, nurse in reverse Trendelenburg.
  - This will encourage venous drainage and reduce cerebral blood volume (CBV) leading to a decrease in ICP.

- Ensure good venous drainage by avoiding endotracheal tube ties. Patients should not have hard collars in place if a neck injury is suspected, as they will be deeply sedated to prevent movement. Leave blocks in place to remind staff about log-rolling.
- Deeply sedate all patients with short-acting hypnotics and opiates such as propofol and alfentanil to a Richmond Agitation Sedation Score (RASS) of −5. Use boluses to prevent/treat small rises in ICP.
- Maintain a CPP of >60 mmHg and an ICP of <20 mmHg. Patients should be euvolaemic before using vasopressors to increase the MAP (and therefore the CPP).
- Ventilate to a $PaCO_2$ of 4.5–5.0 kPa.
    - $PaCO_2$ is an important determinant of cerebral blood flow (CBF).
        - If the $PaCO_2$ is too high (>5.0 kPa), this will cause an increase in CBF and therefore ICP.
        - If the $PaCO_2$ is too low (<4.0 kPa), this will cause a decrease in CBF and can cause ischaemia.
- Maintain a PaO_2 of 11–13 kPa or HbO_2 saturations of >97%.
    - PaO_2 also has an impact on CBF, but obviously has a direct negative impact on cellular function as well.
        - Hypoxia directly increases CBF and therefore ICP.
        - Hypoxia will have a direct negative impact on cellular function and may lead to cerebral oedema.
- Ensure temperature <36.5°C (normothermia).
    - Hyperpyrexia will cause systemic vasodilatation, increased CBF, increased cerebral metabolic rate and increased ICP.
- Maintain a blood glucose of 4–10 mmol/L.
    - Hyperglycaemia will increase cerebral metabolic rate and therefore ICP.

Level 2 Management:

- Ensure ALL Level 1 measures are in place and consider repeat imaging/ surgery.
- Ventilate to a $PaCO_2$ of 4.0–4.5 kPa.
- Use appropriate muscle relaxation, for example atracurium (0.5 mg/kg). If the ICP improves, consider an infusion at 5 mL/hour. (They should already be sedated to RASS of −5!)
- Trial of increasing CPP target to >70 mmHg with noradrenaline. (They should be appropriately filled first! Consider cardiac output monitoring.)
    - This may improve ICP if cerebral autoregulation is intact.

- Consider adding another class of hypnotic agent to deepen sedation, such as midazolam.
- Osmotherapy with hypertonic saline – *This should be a senior decision!*
    - Measure serum osmolarity and plasma Na prior to starting. After starting, measure plasma Na every four hours and monitor fluid balance closely.
    - If plasma Na is >155 mmol/L or calculated plasma osmolality is >320, then hypertonic NaCl is contraindicated. Diabetes insipidus is also a contraindication.
    - Consider a 15-mL bolus of 30% hypertonic saline over 10 minutes. A maximum of 4 boluses can be given in 24 hours.
    - It should be avoided in chronic hyponatraemia or used cautiously if there is a history of cardiac or renal disease.
    - Avoid marked, rapid changes in Na as they may cause rebound cerebral oedema.

Level 3 Management – Requires consultant input:

- Ensure ALL Level 1 and 2 measures are in place and consider repeat imaging/surgery.
- Decompressive craniectomy must be considered to relieve the raised ICP.
    - If performed, it should be performed in conjunction with other medical therapies. It may improve ICP but will not have an effect on pathological cerebral oedema!

Level 4 Management – Requires consultant input:

- Ensure ALL Level 1 and 2 measures are in place and consider repeat imaging. In some occasions, Level 3 may not be appropriate and Level 4 may be performed instead.
- Trial of thiopentone (an intravenous barbiturate hypnotic agent that suppresses cerebral metabolic activity); if 250-mg bolus dose improves CPP, consider thiopentone infusion 4–8 mg/kg/hr.
    - Aim for cerebral burst suppression; this will require specialist monitoring.
- Therapeutic hypothermia.
    - This should only be considered in rescue scenarios with specific cases with severe resistant raised ICP. There is some evidence that this may be harmful so this should not be considered lightly!

KEY LEARNING POINTS

- Management of a potential traumatic brain injury requires a thorough, structured 'ABC' approach.
- Call for help early, as patients may deteriorate rapidly, and require specialist management, such as intubation.
- Avoid even single episodes of hypoxia and hypotension, as these can have detrimental effects on overall outcome!
- If ICP monitoring is not available, assume the ICP is at least 20 mmHg and start Level 1 treatments before arriving at a neuro-surgical centre!

FURTHER READING

Brain Trauma Foundation. "Guidelines for the Management of Severe Traumatic Brain Injury." *Journal of Neurotrauma* 24, Supplement 1 (2007): S1–S116.

Girling, Keith. "Management of Head Injury in the Intensive Care Unit." *Continuing Education in Anaesthesia Critical Care & Pain* 4, no. 2 (April 2004): 52–56.

Helmy, Adel, Marcela Vizcaychipi, and Arun K. Gupta. "Traumatic Brain Injury: Intensive Care Management." *British Journal of Anaesthesia* 99, no. 1 (July 2007): 32–42.

16

Initial management of the patient with burns

KAREN MEACHER AND NITIN ARORA

'Hi, we've had a pre-alert from ambulance control and are expecting multiple patients who've been in a house fire to be brought in, in the next 10 minutes. The ED registrar has requested that you attend if possible to help with the initial assessment of one of the patients'.

Whilst the Emergency Department is more than capable of managing burns patients as they come through the door, patients with significant burns will need to be cared for in an intensive care setting. However, depending on how local services are organised, it is possible you may be involved in the initial management of these patients.

Burns and thermal injuries can be devastating and complex, but like most (all!) things you will deal with in critical care, a structured approach means you will not miss anything important.

THE BASICS OF BURNS

A burn is an injury to the skin and tissues that is usually thought of as being caused by heat (thermal) but can also be caused by cold, chemicals, electricity, friction and radiation.

Thermal burn injuries can be caused by hot liquids and steam, contact from hot objects, and fire or explosive materials. There are two elements that need to be considered when assessing burns:

1. Depth
   - Erythema (aka 'first degree') e.g. sunburn
     - Damage to superficial epidermis only
     - Red and painful
     - No blistering (epidermis intact)
     - **Not included when assessing size of burn**
   - Partial thickness (aka 'second degree')
     - Damage to the epidermis
     - Red or mottled
     - Exquisitely painful due to exposed nerve endings
     - Weeping, oedematous, blistered skin
   - Full thickness (aka 'third degree')
     - Damage to both epidermis and dermis (and potentially subcutaneous tissues)
     - May appear: charred, red, dark and leathery, or pale and waxy
     - Tends to be painless but patients may complain of constant dull pain
     - Skin is dry with minimal swelling
2. Size
   - Extent of burn is expressed as a percentage of body surface area (BSA)
   - Wallace Rule of Nines
     - Useful method of estimating extent of burns

- Adult body is broken down into areas that are multiples of 9% BSA
- Paediatric variation takes account of children's heads being a proportionately bigger component of BSA
- Area of patient's (not your!) palm and fingers is roughly 1% of BSA
- Lund–Browder charts
  - Paper based chart that may be available in your local ED
  - More useful for paediatric patients as it gives a variable % BSA depending on the patient's age

The functions of skin include protection (a barrier against infection and mechanical damage), immunity, temperature regulation and fluid regulation. The greater the % BSA affected by a burn, the more significant the consequences to the patient. A greater than 30% BSA results in a systemic inflammatory response due to the release of cytokines and other inflammatory mediators. Thus, estimation of % BSA is vital to help determine what the best management of the patient will be.

It is also important to get as much history of how the burn occurred as possible (as well as the standard AMPLE history) either from the patient or from the paramedics who have transferred them from the scene of injury.

- What circumstance caused the injury? e.g. house fire, RTC, explosion
- Was the patient trapped in an enclosed space, and if so, for how long?
- Are there any associated injuries?

Be aware that all types of burns are initially managed according to ATLS-type principles because they are frequently associated with trauma, e.g. have been involved in an RTC where the vehicle subsequently set alight.

You have come down to resus and are ready and waiting as three members of the same family are brought in by paramedics. You are directed to assess an adult male who is wearing a cervical collar and is triple immobilised on a spinal board and receiving 15 L O_2 via mask with reservoir bag. He is asking how his son and wife are whilst intermittently coughing. Paramedics tell you that he jumped from a first-floor window holding his son in his arms and landed on his back. They report they have noticed burn injuries affecting all four limbs but they have not investigated this in any detail. It was reported at the scene that he and his son had been trapped in his son's bedroom for 20 minutes before he managed to break the window open wide enough to jump out. What do you do next?

ASSESSMENT

Assessment is structured according to Advanced Trauma Life Support (ATLS) principles of primary and secondary surveys; please refer to Chapter 14 for further information. The basic structure is

- Airway + C-spine control
- Breathing
- Circulation
- Disability
- Exposure

A more detailed explanation can be found in Chapter 14, but there are specific considerations to assessing burn injuries. Remember that it is important not to focus on (and get distracted by) the obvious injuries, especially in the context of multiple traumas.

General considerations:

- Apply high-flow oxygen via mask with reservoir bag.
- Remove all clothes (unless stuck to the skin) and jewellery (subsequent tissue swelling may cause a tourniquet).
- Burns should be dressed with cling film as soon as possible.
- Ensure the patient is kept warm with sheets and blankets (vulnerable to hypothermia).
- Bloods: group and save (G&S), arterial blood gas, full blood count (FBC), urea and electrolytes (U&Es), clotting, glucose.
- Imaging: chest X-ray.

AIRWAY AND BREATHING

Smoke inhalation injury results from exposure to the harmful gases, vapours and particles in smoke occurring due to combustion of materials. It can result in thermal injury, respiratory injury and toxic injury (or a combination), and has a high associated mortality.

THERMAL INJURY

Thermal injury to the upper airways will result in tissue oedema and swelling, eventually leading to airway obstruction. If you have any concern that a patient has sustained a thermal airway injury, then escalate to a senior for assessment for early intubation of the patient. Indications for *immediate* intubation are

- Decreased consciousness, confusion or agitation
- Hoarse voice or stridor
- Respiratory distress, inadequate respiratory effort or hypoxaemia
- Impending or clinically apparent airway obstruction

In the alert, appropriate and talking patient, points from the history or clinical examination that may raise your suspicions are

- Voice changes (ask patient if voice sounds normal to them)
- Burns to face or neck
- Singed eyebrows or nasal hairs
- Soot deposits in nose or mouth
- Coughing up black (carbonaceous) sputum
- History of being confined in a burning building
- History of loss of consciousness at scene
- History of death of another person at scene

Not all patients with an inhalation injury require intubation but as swelling and oedema continue in the first 24 to 36 hours after injury, there is often a low-threshold for intubation.

Intubation should be supervised or performed by the most appropriately skilled and experienced clinician available, which is often the general anaesthetic consultant or ICU consultant on call. The endotracheal tube is left uncut so that subsequent facial and airway swelling do not dislodge the tube.

Remember to pass a nasogastric feeding tube at the same time, which will enable early feeding. If missed, it may be impossible to pass a feeding tube (due to swelling of soft tissues) for a prolonged period, and TPN may be necessary.

RESPIRATORY INJURY

Particulate matter (soot) is inhaled into the respiratory tree, where it causes localised irritation and swelling as well as mechanical obstruction of the airways. This results in a cascade of inflammatory mediators and the end result is an ARDS-like picture with significant ventilation/perfusion mismatch, hypoxia and tissue necrosis. Indications for early intubation and bronchoscopy with washout are as above.

TOXIC INJURY

A person confined in a burning building is vulnerable to hypoxic and toxic injury. First, the fire consumes the oxygen in the local environment and so they end up breathing a hypoxic (FiO_2 <0.21) gas mix. As a result, they will have potentially experienced significant tissue hypoxia.

Additionally, they have inhaled a number of toxic chemicals. The chemical composition of smoke is dependent on the material being burned and how much oxygen is available to aid combustion. Two important toxins to be aware of are carbon monoxide (CO) and hydrogen cyanide (HCN), as these will perpetuate tissue hypoxia despite the patient no longer being in a hypoxic environment.

- Carbon monoxide
    - 240 times affinity for haemoglobin over O_2, and so reduces O_2 uptake
    - Causes a left-shift of the oxygen dissociation curve, so less O_2 delivered to tissues
    - Competitively inhibits binding of O_2 with mitochondrial enzymes and impairs cellular utilization of O_2
    - Assume CO poisoning in any patients removed from enclosed fires
    - Treat with application of high-flow O_2 until levels normalise (FiO_2 1.0 if intubated)
- Hydrogen cyanide
    - Bonds with and structurally alters mitochondrial enzymes causing impaired cellular respiration
    - 20 times more toxic than CO
    - Unable to easily measure CN^- levels (only centre in UK is Cardiff, with a two-week turnaround!)
    - Consider administration of antidote, hydroxocobalamin, in patients with significantly raised lactate, raised anion gap acidosis, reduced arteriovenous O_2 gradient and history of smoke inhalation injury for whom all other causes of a raised lactate have been addressed

CIRCULATION

Fluid resuscitation and maintenance

Patients with burns have potentially very high fluid requirements due to a combination of massive fluid shifts and evaporation due to loss of skin barrier function.

- Termed 'burn shock'
- Fluid resuscitation indicated in >15% BSA (>10% BSA children and elderly)
- Minimum 2 large bore (14G or 16G) peripheral IV access
  - Site preferentially through unburned skin
  - May need to be sited through burn if injury extensive
- Intra-arterial pressure monitoring advantageous
- Urinary catheter

The Parkland formula is used to guide crystalloid fluid resuscitation requirements for patients with burns injuries in the first 24 hours.

Volume of fluid required = 4 mL × patient weight (kg) × % BSA

e.g. 80-kg patient with 40% burns = 4 mL × 80 × 40 = 12,800 mL

- Half given in the first eight hours since the burn was sustained (not arrival in ED)
- Second half over the subsequent 16 hours
- e.g. if injury at 10 am and now 2 pm, they would need:
  - 6400 mL of crystalloid (e.g. compound sodium lactate solution) over the next four hours, i.e. 1600 mL/hr
  - 6400 mL over the subsequent 16 hours, i.e. 400 mL/hr

However, the Parkland formula is a *guide* not a rule. Some patients may require more fluids, some less. When you factor in additional fluid or blood product resuscitation due to trauma, you can see how it is not quite as neat a calculation as you would wish it could be. Strive to use hourly urine output to fine tune fluid requirements by aiming for 0.5 mL/kg/hr (1.0 mL/kg/hr in children).

CIRCUMFERENTIAL BURNS

A circumferential burn is a burn that extends around a limb or the torso. It creates a band of scar tissue (eschar) that, as the tissues swell due to oedema formation, exerts a tourniquet effect.

- Neck – airway obstruction, impaired cerebral perfusion, raised ICP
- Chest – reduced chest expansion compromising respiration/ventilation
- Abdomen – abdominal compartment syndrome, organ failure
- Limbs – muscle compartment syndrome, limb ischaemia

Any circumferential burn should be immediately referred to surgery for consideration of escharotomy.

DISABILITY

Assess GCS, pupillary reflexes, and rule out traumatic brain injury. Check blood glucose.

EXPOSURE

Examine the whole of the patient's body (do not forget the back), then cover the patient. Burns patients may lose heat rapidly, causing them to become hypothermic. Raising the room temperature or radiant heat is often required.

ONGOING MANAGEMENT

Once a patient has been assessed, they need to be cared for in an appropriate environment. For less significant burn injuries, that may be the hospital they have presented to; severe burn injuries will need to be transferred to a specialist burn centre. The British Burn Association offers guidance as to whether a patient should be discussed with specialists or referred to a specialist centre, depending on five criteria:

- % BSA
- Depth (all full thickness burns)
- Site (all circumferential burns; burns to hands, feet or perineum)
- Mechanism (all non-thermal burn injuries; non-accidental injuries)
- Other factors (major trauma; significant co-morbidities; pregnancy)

KEY LEARNING POINTS

- Management of burns requires a thorough, structured 'ABC' approach.
- Call for help early, as patients may deteriorate rapidly, and require specialist management, such as intubation.
- Do not cut the endotracheal tube. Ensure NG is passed early.
- Maintain adequate fluid balance: this may need large amounts of crystalloids.
- Any burns patient that needs intubation should go to a burns centre.

FURTHER READING

American College of Surgeons. *Advanced Trauma Life Support Student Course Manual*. 9th edition. Chicago: American College of Surgeons, 2012.

British Burn Association. www.britishburnassociation.org.

Mersey Burns—Free app for most phone platforms that calculates % BSA and Parkland Formula. http://merseyburns.com.

National Network for Burn Care. *National Burn Care Referral Guidance*. London: British Burn Association, 2012. www.britishburnassociation .org/downloads/National_Burn_Care_Referral_Guidance_-_5.2.12.pdf.

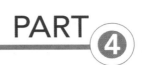

PART 4

DRUGS

17

Analgesia, sedation and muscle relaxation

HOZEFA EBRAHIM

Mrs Smith has been intubated for ventilation on the ICU. She was hypoxic, secondary to a severe pneumonia. The nurses ask you which drugs you'd like to use to sedate this patient. How do you choose which drugs to prescribe?

INTRODUCTION

Sedation, analgesia and muscle relaxation are commonly used on the intensive care unit. Patients may have post-operative pain, need opiates for tube tolerance, or sedation to cope with the discomfort of multiple interventions we carry out. Muscle relaxation is mainly used to aid difficult ventilation. Whilst the intention is always to aid the treatment and recovery of the patient, we must remember that these potent drugs also have adverse effects.

ANALGESIA

Analgesia must be titrated to the needs of the individual. Most ICU patients require some form of analgesia. Patients may present with acute or chronic pain issues, or a combination of both.

Paracetamol is generally a safe analgesic and is given through both enteral and parenteral routes. IV paracetamol reaches the site of action much more quickly then the enteral route, and is argued to have an analgesic effect similar to 10 mg of IM morphine. When given four times a day, a therapeutic concentration builds up in the bloodstream and provides a better clinical outcome. It is worth noting that paracetamol may mask pyrexia in certain individuals. Paracetamol should also be used with caution in patients with liver impairment. Patients with a weight under 50 kg should be given a reduced regular dose.

Non-steroidal anti-inflammatory drugs (NSAIDs) are utilised less frequently in ICU. Whilst they provide good analgesia in young surgical patients who are otherwise healthy, they are associated with a higher degree of gastro-intestinal haemorrhage, renal impairment and ischaemic cardiac events. All of these complications are common in ICU. Some surgeons believe NSAIDs also increase the post-surgical bleed rate.

Many different types of opioids are used in ICU. Morphine and fentanyl are often used in patient-controlled analgesia (PCA). Morphine, fentanyl, alfentanil and remifentanil are all used in infusions. All have their pros and cons, and different hospitals have their own preferences. As well as providing analgesia, they also offer a degree of sedation. Opioids can also be used as patches, lozenges and subcutaneous routes, but these are less common. As a rough rule, most intubated and ventilated patients will require some form of low-rate infused opioids. Always remember to titrate the drug to effect.

As these drugs make up a large proportion of ICU management (and ICU problems), it is important to know some detailed pharmacology. Opioids are weak bases, and therefore dissociate into ionised and un-ionised forms in solution. Diffusion and absorption are dependent on the un-ionised fraction, which is in turn dependent on local pH. Some drugs undergo *first pass metabolism* in the gut wall and liver, and this depends upon a number of patient factors. Lipid solubility and protein binding determine how the drug is transported, released and available to tissues within the body. Both these properties are dependent on patient health. Hepatic and renal function determines how these drugs are metabolised and eliminated from the body. In summary, the same dose of the same drug can have a varied effect on two similar patients. This is why is it extremely important to titrate opioids to effect, and continually monitor and adjust therapy.

CONTEXT-SENSITIVE HALF-LIFE

This term is given to illustrate how the half-life of a drug may depend upon the context in which it is used. Most commonly, we refer to the increased half-life of a drug in the *context* of a prolonged infusion. For example, the longer fentanyl is used in infusion, as bodily tissues become increasingly saturated in the drug, the elimination half-life increases. This is why fentanyl is not frequently used to sedate patients in ICU (Table 17.1).

It is essential to titrate these infusions to effect. The required rate differs depending upon age, weight, pathology, renal and hepatic function, and many other factors.

An increasingly common form of pain control comes in the form of regional anaesthesia. Epidurals have been used for many years following surgical procedures. However, due to lessons learnt from peri-operative physicians, other regional techniques have come into vogue to reduce the adverse effects of epidurals. These include single-shot blocks (e.g. femoral, sciatic, intercostal, axillary), as well as in-dwelling catheters (e.g. rectus sheath blocks). The insertion of these blocks must be performed by an experienced practitioner. The drugs used in these regional analgesic techniques are local anaesthetics, such as bupivacaine. These drugs are not injected intravenously. Be aware of the maximum safe dose of local anaesthetics. Even when injected into soft tissues, they have the ability to be absorbed quickly enough to cause cardiac and neurological complications.

SEDATION

Opiates have a sedating effect as well as analgesic properties. However, we also use specific sedative agents (also known as hypnotics). The most common are propofol and midazolam, but others such as thiopentone (neuroscience units), dexmedetomidine and clonidine are also seen.

These drugs may be used as boluses or infusions, though infusions are much more common. As explained above, sedatives should be titrated to effect. This is explained in Table 17.2, which describes the characteristics of several sedatives.

Table 17.1 Properties of different opioids in ICU

	Morphine	Fentanyl	Alfentanil	Remifentanil
Dosing information and typical infusion regimes	Infusion: 1 mg·mL^{-1} in 50 mL syringe Rate: 0–10 mL·hr^{-1}	Infusion: 50 mcg·mL^{-1} in 50 mL syringe Rate: 0–5 mL·hr^{-1}	Infusion: 500 mcg·mL^{-1} in 50 mL syringe Rate: 0–5 mL·hr^{-1}	Infusion: 100 mg·mL^{-1} in 50 mL syringe Rate: 0–5 mL·hr^{-1}
Elimination half-life (min)	170	190	100	5
Clearance (mL·min^{-1}·kg^{-1})	16	1	6	40
Volume of distribution (L·kg^{-1})	3.5	4.0	0.6	0.3
Protein binding (%)	35	83	90	70
pKa	8.0	8.4	6.5	7.1
Ionisation at pH 7.4 (%)	77	91	11	32
Lipid solubility (octanol:water coefficient)	1	600	90	20

(*Continued*)

Table 17.1 (*Continued*) Properties of different opioids in ICU

	Morphine	Fentanyl	Alfentanil	Remifentanil
Advantages	Cheap Long acting analgesia Euphoria Properties well known	Less hypotension than other opiates	Short acting	Excellent for weaning Excellent tube tolerance No accumulation in hepatic/renal failure Ultra-short acting
Disadvantages	Active metabolites accumulate in hepatic/renal failure	Increased context-sensitive half-life Varied absorption with fevers (increased)	More haemodynamic and respiratory compromise when compared to morphine and fentanyl	Expensive Enhanced haemodynamic and respiratory compromise

Note: These figures are meant to illustrate a trend. Please apply caution as figures may differ slightly from text to text.

Table 17.2 Properties of different sedatives on ICU

	Propofol	Midazolam	Dexmedetomidine	Thiopentone
Dosing information and typical infusion regimes	1% or 2% neat. 50 mL syringe. Up to 20 mL·hr⁻¹	1–2 mg·mL⁻¹ Up to 10 mL·hr⁻¹		25 mg·mL⁻¹ 0–20 mL·hr⁻¹
Elimination half-life (hr)	4–7	1.7–2.6	2–3	7–17
Clearance (mL·min⁻¹·kg⁻¹)	20–30	6–11	10–30	3–4
Volume of distribution (L·kg⁻¹)	2–10	1–2	2–3	1.5–3
Advantages	Short acting	Safe in bolus form Cheap	Very short acting Excellent for weaning Allows awake weaning Has analgesic effect No respiratory depression	Good seizure control
Disadvantages	Hypotension Propofol infusion syndrome (paediatrics mainly)	Drug interactions Accumulation in renal failure	Expensive Not approved for use widely in UK	Very long acting

Note: These figures are to illustrate a trend. Please apply caution as figures may differ slightly from text to text.

TITRATION OF ANALGESIA AND SEDATION

Too little sedation and the patient will experience unpleasant events. Too much, and they will develop a host of side effects. Similarly, titration of *analgesia* is equally important. Various scoring systems exist to gauge the depth of sedation of an ICU patient. Scoring systems also exist to measure a patient's pain level. Infusion rates can be increased and decreased in order to titrate drug levels to the desired effect for individuals.

The Richmond Agitation-Sedation Scale (RASS) is a scoring system used in ICU to gauge a patient's sedation level. The scores range from $+4$ to -5. We aim to maintain patients at a RASS of -1 to 0 (Table 17.3).

Patients are frequently over-sedated, leading to prolonged waking times, a worry about potential intracranial events (with subsequent CT scans, etc.), delirium and prolonged ICU stay. Much evidence now guides us to practice 'sedation holds'. Every morning, sedation infusions are stopped, and the sedation score of the patient is assessed continuously (unless there

Table 17.3 Richmond Agitation-Sedation Scale

		Richmond Agitation-Sedation Scale (RASS)
+4	Combative	Violent – immediate danger to staff or self
+3	Very agitated	Pulls or removes tubes or catheters – aggressive
+2	Agitated	Frequent, non-purposeful movement, fights ventilator
+1	Restless	Anxious, apprehensive but movements not aggressive or vigorous
0	Alert and calm	
−1	Drowsy	Not fully alert, but easily responds to voice – focuses for >10 secs
−2	Light sedation	Briefly responds to voice – focuses for <10 secs
−3	Moderate sedation	Movement or eye opening to voice – but no eye contact or obeying commands
−4	Deep sedation	No response to voice, but moves to painful stimulus
−5	Unrousable	No response to voice or painful stimulus

Table 17.4 Contraindications to sedation holds

Absolute Contraindications	Relative Contraindication
Continuous muscle paralysis agent	Moderate ventilatory requirements
Extreme ventilatory requirements	High FiO$_2$
Very high FiO$_2$	Imminent procedure such as theatre,
Known high ICP	tracheostomy, etc.
Withdrawal of curative treatment	

is a contraindication to stopping sedation – see Table 17.4). Infusions are recommenced only once the patient has reached their required level of wakefulness. This method prevents us from saturating tissues with excessive amounts of sedative agents. This practice has been shown to reduce morbidity and mortality, decrease length of stay on ICU and decrease delirium rates.

MUSCLE RELAXATION

Most ICU patients do not require continuous muscle relaxation. Indeed, we prefer patients to maintain their own respiratory effort in many cases. Muscle relaxation is used when we intubate patients, and sometimes when ventilation is particularly difficult. Such examples include a patient with severe ARDS with high ventilatory pressures. Nursing staff may describe these patients as 'fighting the ventilator'.

On initial intubation of a patient, a muscle is used. This may be suxamethonium (a depolarising muscle relaxant) or a non-depolarising agent such as rocuronium or atracurium. When intubating typical ICU patients, the primary aim is to obtain intubating conditions quickly and safely. With regard to muscle relaxants, the quicker agents are suxamethonium and rocuronium. The advantages of suxamethonium are that it is tried and tested, works within 45 seconds, and is readily available. The disadvantages are that it causes muscle pain, increases potassium levels marginally, is associated with 'sux apnoea' and anaphylaxis, and raises intracranial/intra-ocular pressure. The advantages of rocuronium are that it is also readily available and acts quickly. However, it does not cause muscle pain. The disadvantage (but also an advantage) is that it lasts a long time – approximately 40 minutes. It is also associated with anaphylaxis.

MANAGING SEDATION FOR MRS SMITH

Mrs Smith has already been anaesthetised in order to intubate her and commence ventilation. For this purpose, the ICU doctors will have chosen an *induction agent*, most likely either propofol or thiopentone. They will have used a *muscle relaxant* in order to relax the vocal cords to facilitate passing an endotracheal tube, either rocuronium or suxamethonium. In addition, they would have used a fast acting opiate to obtund the cardiac reflex to intubation (if her haemodynamics allowed this); the drugs of choice are often fentanyl or alfentanil.

Following induction of anaesthesia, she requires sedation and analgesia to keep her tolerant of the interventions needed: intubation and ventilation. Common choices are infusions of propofol with alfentanil. Propofol is used because it is relatively short acting and predictable. It is easily titrated. Alfentanil is similarly easy to titrate, is quick acting and wears off quickly. Unlike fentanyl, following prolonged infusion, it does not show a context-sensitive prolonged half-life. An ongoing muscle relaxant is unlikely to be needed unless Mrs Smith is particularly difficult to ventilate or oxygenate.

KEY LEARNING POINTS

- Analgesia, anxiolysis, sedation and muscle relaxants can be given by infusion or as boluses.
- Most ICU patients require some form of analgesia and/or sedation during their stay.
- Prolonged infusions take longer to wear off.
- Over-sedation can contribute to delirium.
- Be aware of ICU-induced opioid dependence and withdrawal.

FURTHER READING

Smith, Tim, Colin Pinnock, Ted Lin, and Robert Jones (eds). *Fundamentals of Anaesthesia*, 3rd edition. Cambridge: Cambridge University Press, 2009.

- Chapter 6: Hypnotics and Intravenous Anaesthetic Agents
- Chapter 7: Analgesic Drugs
- Chapter 8: Neuromuscular Blocking Agents

It is advisable to refer to the *British National Formulary* constantly whenever prescribing anything other than the very common prescriptions. *The Oxford Handbook of Anaesthesia* is a valuable resource to consult. Both publications are available as digital versions downloadable onto a smartphone.

All trainees must be familiar with local guidelines. Deviations from standard concentrations and infusion rates can risk confusion in the workplace.

18

Drugs that work on the heart

RACHEL HOWARTH AND ANDREW HAUGHTON

Mr Smith in Bed 10, admitted with sepsis secondary to community acquired pneumonia, remains hypotensive. His blood pressure is only 80/40 mmHg despite receiving 1500 mL of fluid in the last two hours. He is anuric, and becoming increasingly drowsy. What do you want to do?

This chapter will focus on medications that affect the cardiovascular system, in particular drugs affecting blood pressure. Anti-dysrhythmic drugs will not be discussed as these are explained in Chapter 31.

BLOOD PRESSURE

In general terms, we may need to either increase or decrease a patient's blood pressure. It is important to remember that although the drugs' effects are exerted on blood pressure, it is often end organ perfusion that is the primary concern. In this respect, monitor the patient holistically and avoid merely chasing the 'perfect' blood pressure number.

Firstly, we need to consider the factors that influence blood pressure. In simple terms, the heart is a pump, which can vary its rate and strength of contraction. The blood is being pumped around a circulation that essentially consists of three parts:

1. The arterial system, of which the pressure determines the supply pressure to organs. The pressure here also influences how much the heart empties during each contraction.
2. The capillary system, which is large and low pressure, through which individual organs flow, is therefore governed by the feeding pressure.
3. The venous system, which is large and in which the pressure determines the rate of flow back to the heart.

$$\text{Cardiac output} = \text{heart rate} \times \text{stroke volume}$$

And cardiac output is proportional to blood pressure:

$$\text{Mean arterial pressure} = \text{cardiac output} \times \text{systemic vascular resistance}$$

INCREASING BLOOD PRESSURE

Using the above equations, it can be seen that blood pressure can be increased by increasing heart rate or by increasing stroke volume (provided increasing one does not decrease the other at the same time!).

What is perhaps less obvious is that blood pressure can also be increased by increasing vascular tone – that is, by decreasing the arterial volume. This has the potential disadvantage that by increasing tone and therefore also blood pressure, blood flow (i.e. cardiac output) is actually reduced.

At any given time we rarely have accurate measures of all of these variables, and this is why it is important to remember that blood pressure alone should not be a target. If in doubt, assess clinically whether the patient is improving (e.g. by using urine output or lactate levels as markers of perfusion).

The discussion of the drugs, which follows, describes the general principles of their actions, but individual patients' responses will vary depending on their underlying physiology. Whenever you initiate treatment with any of these drugs, consider carefully what you want to achieve. Then, assess the patient response and be prepared to be wrong and to change the drug!

To help to categorise different medication actions, the following terms are useful:

- *Inotrope* – a substance that increases cardiac muscle contractility (in almost all cases by increasing cardiac intracellular calcium levels)
- *Chronotrope* – a substance that affects heart rate
- *Vasopressor* – a substance that increases vascular tone and resistance

DRUGS

- *Adrenaline* – a naturally occurring catecholamine, which has a potent effect on beta receptors 1 and 2 in all areas. As such, it is a positive inotrope with a mixed effect on vascular tone depending on the tissues.
- *Noradrenaline* – a naturally occurring catecholamine that is active at alpha receptors. It causes intense vasoconstriction in most arterioles, and has some moderate inotropic actions.
- *Dopamine* – a catecholamine precursor of the above that has some properties of both. It also works on specific dopamine receptors, which cause splanchnic vasodilatation and diuresis. Its effects at alpha and beta receptors are partly dose-dependent, with the beta effect predominating at low doses and the alpha effect at higher doses.
- *Dobutamine* – a synthetic catecholamine that is used mainly as an inotrope. It also has significant chronotropic effects.
- *Digoxin* – although now usually used for rate control in atrial fibrillation, it was previously used as a treatment for heart failure, due to its inotropic actions, secondary to its influence at sodium potassium channels, rather than to any beta-agonist effects.
- *Metaraminol* – a sympathomimetic adrenoceptor agonist that has both direct and indirect alpha-1 agonism resulting in peripheral vasoconstriction.
- *Glucagon* – primarily causes an increase in blood sugar levels, but it also has inotropic effects, which are independent of beta receptors. This makes it a useful drug in cases of beta-blocker overdose.
- *Phosphodiesterase inhibitors* – by reducing the breakdown of cAMP, these drugs help to increase calcium levels within cells, and thus in the heart they act as inotropes. They have a broad spectrum of effects, depending on which type of enzymes they tend to inhibit. Theophylline is mainly a bronchodilator, whereas enoximone and milrinone are mainly cardiac inotropes. However, all will have an element of action in all phosphodiesterase enzyme subsets.

DECREASING BLOOD PRESSURE

This is mainly achieved by vasodilatation and slowing of the heart rate. Hypertension is a less common problem in critical care than hypotension, and unless the blood pressure is very high, it is often not necessary to aggressively treat in the short term in unstable patients.

When assessing the hypertensive patient, it is also worth considering the potential causes, e.g. pain, anxiety, and the need for anxiolytics and analgesics.

DRUGS

- *Glyceryl trinitrate (GTN)* – a vasodilator that in low doses affects mainly veins, and at higher doses also affects arterioles. It lowers blood pressure and leaves cardiac output unaltered or moderately reduced.
- *Hydralazine* – an arteriolar vasodilator that lowers vascular resistance and therefore decreases blood pressure, but can cause a reflex tachycardia.
- *Labetalol* – a beta and alpha blocker, so at the same time as reducing vascular resistance, it also blocks any reflex tachycardia. Therefore, it will reduce blood pressure and cardiac output simultaneously.
- *Phentolamine* – This is an alpha 1 and 2 blocker, so it causes vasodilation and some inotropic effects. It reduces the blood pressure with an increased cardiac output.

Many of these infusions can only be given via a central venous line and require invasive arterial monitoring.

HOW TO USE THESE MEDICATIONS IN A CLINICAL SETTING

In a hypotensive patient, first, always ensure adequate filling pressures, perhaps by assessing the effects of a fluid bolus. In a hypertensive patient, assess the need for anxiolytics or analgesia. Always make sure that the reading is accurate. If this is an invasive blood pressure reading, check whether the transducers are at the correct level, whether it has been zeroed, and whether it is a good arterial waveform. Generally, invasive blood pressure monitoring is needed to enable real-time titration of inotrope/vasopressor infusions. The following are examples of typical doses and dilutions in our unit.

- *In a septic, vasodilated patient:* noradrenaline, 4 mg made up to 40 mL with 5% glucose started at 5 mL/hour and titrated up or down against response.
- *In a patient with a reduced cardiac output:* dobutamine, 250 mg made up to 50 mL with normal saline, started at 5 mL/hour and titrated up or down according to response. If the response to dobutamine is not adequate, consider adrenaline, 5 mg made up to 50 mL with normal saline, started at 5 mL/hour and titrated up or down.
- *In a hypotensive patient after beta-blocker overdose:* consider glucagon, 20 mg made up to 40 mL with 5% glucose, infused at 0–20 mL/hour according to response.
- *In a hypertensive patient, with normal or high heart rate:* consider labetalol, which is available as 100 mg in 20 mL, given neat at a rate of 5–30 mL/hour according to response.
- *In a hypertensive patient in whom beta blockers are contraindicated:* glyceryl trinitrate (GTN), premixed at 1 mg/mL, given at a rate of 1–20 mL/hour.

WHAT DO YOU DO IN RESPONSE TO THE NURSE'S QUESTION?

Remember your ABCDE approach when assessing the patient, and to seek senior help as needed.

A. Is the airway patent? This is a concern if the patient is becoming increasingly drowsy – are they likely to require intubation?
B. What is their respiratory rate, and oxygen saturations? What respiratory support are they already requiring, given their presentation with community-acquired pneumonia?
C. What is their heart rate, blood pressure and capillary refill time? What is their fluid status? What is their overall fluid balance?
D. What is their temperature, GCS, blood glucose?
E. Exposure and complete examination – to assess for any evidence of blood/fluid loss.

Ensure the patient has an arterial line sited, for invasive blood pressure monitoring. For their blood pressure management, the patient has already received 1500 mL in the last two hours. After assessing fluid status, providing there is no clinical evidence of fluid overload and if clinically they appear fluid deplete, it may be worthwhile to try a further 500 mL fluid challenge. However, this patient is highly likely to need vasopressor/inotropic support and in the first instance should be commenced on a metaraminol infusion (20 mg metaraminol in 40 mL 0.9% NaCl), which can be given peripherally at an infusion rate up to 20 mL/hr. If their metaraminol requirements are escalating or he remains hypotensive, he will require central venous access and commencing on a noradrenaline infusion. In this case, cardiac output monitoring is likely to be useful to guide further management.

Finally, ensure the patient is receiving appropriate treatment and antibiotic therapy for their underlying pneumonia.

KEY LEARNING POINTS

- Always check the accuracy of the reading.
- In a hypotensive patient, ensure you have checked for adequate filling pressures, perhaps by assessing the effects of a fluid bolus.
- In patients with escalating vasopressor or inotropic requirements, the use of cardiac output monitoring is useful to guide decisions on further management.
- In a hypertensive patient, ensure you have assessed the need for anxiolytics or analgesia.

FURTHER READING

Müllner, Marcus, Bernhard Urbanek, Christof Havel, Heidrun Losert, Gunnar Gamper, and Harald Herkner. "Vasopressors for Shock." *Cochrane Database of Systematic Reviews*, no. 3 (July 2004): CD003709.

Rhodes, Andrew, Laura E. Evans, Waleed Alhazzani, Mitchell M. Levy, Massimo Antonelli, Ricard Ferrer, Anand Kumar, Jonathan E. Sevransky, Charles M. Sprung, Mark E. Nunnally, Bram Rochwerg, Gordon D. Rubenfeld, Derek C. Angus, Djillali Annane, Richard J. Beale, Geoffrey J. Bellinghan, Gordon R. Bernard, Jean-Daniel Chiche, Craig Coopersmith, Daniel P. De Backer, Craig J. French, Seitaro Fujishima, Herwig Gerlach, Jorge Luis Hidalgo, Steven M. Hollenberg, Alan E. Jones, Dilip R. Karnad, Ruth M. Kleinpell, Younsuck Koh, Thiago Costa Lisboa, Flavia Machado,

John J. Marini, John C. Marshall, John E. Mazuski, Lauralyn A. McIntyre, Anthony S. McLean, Sangeeta Mehta, Rui P. Moreno, John Myburgh, Paolo Navalesi, Osamu Nishida, Tiffany M. Osborn, Anders Perner, Colleen M. Plunkett, Marco Ranieri, Christa A. Schorr, Maureen A. Seckel, Christopher W. Seymour, Lisa Shieh, Khalid A. Shukri, Steven Q. Simpson, Mervyn Singer, B. Taylor Thompson, Sean R. Townsend, Thomas van der Poll, Jean-Louis Vincent, W. Joost Wiersinga, Janice L. Zimmerman, and R. Phillip Dellinger. "Surviving Sepsis Campaign: International Guidelines for Management of Sepsis and Septic Shock: 2016." *Critical Care Medicine* 45, no. 3 (March 2017): 486–552.

Yentis, Steven, Nicholas Hirsch, and Gary Smith. *Anaesthesia and Intensive Care A-Z: An Encyclopaedia of Principles and Practice*, 5th ed. Edinburgh: Churchill Livingstone, 2013.

19

Nutrition and fluids in intensive care

BEN SLATER

Nutrition is easily overlooked in the daily review of critically ill patients but is crucial to their ability to survive acute illness. Malnutrition is common in the critically ill and leads to reduced muscle bulk and power, which can lead to impaired respiratory and cardiac function, immune dysfunction, anaemia, gut mucosal atrophy, poor wound healing, reduced cognitive function, poor sleep pattern and depression.

A multidisciplinary approach to nutritional support in ICU is standard with thorough assessment by dieticians and collateral history from relatives.

Oral feeding is preferable to avoid the bypassing of innate gastrointestinal reflexes, which naturally facilitate digestion and absorption of nutrients.

However, in critically ill patients, swallowing is often inadequate due to artificial airway, sedation or underlying illness in which case nasoenteral feeding should be commenced.

This does require intact gastrointestinal function, which may be impaired in the presence of: mechanical or pseudo-obstruction, small bowel fistula, malabsorption or intractable diarrhoea.

That being the case, parenteral nutrition may be totally or partially indicated.

Current evidence base does not support early parenteral nutrition (before one week) over late parenteral nutrition (after one week) in critically ill patients. Initial malfunctioning gastrointestinal function normally resolves within a week of introducing enteral nutrition and prokinetics, avoiding the risks of parenteral nutrition.

Enteral feeding can be provided by nasogastric (NG), post-pyloric, nasojejunal (NJ) or percutaneous gastrostomy tube. Post-pyloric feeding is favoured in those individuals with gastroparesis and may be provided by weighted or 'hooked' (Tiger) tubes with radiological confirmation or endoscopically placed 'double-lumen' NG/NJ tubes.

Parenteral feeding is ideally provided via a peripherally inserted catheter (PIC), peripherally inserted central catheter (PICC) or central venous catheter (CVC).

Screen patients (Malnutrition Universal Screening Tool [MUST]) on admission and weekly thereafter.

Clinical suspicion of malnutrition
Unintentional weight loss, fragile skin, poor wound healing, apathy, wasted muscles, poor appetite, altered taste and sensation, impaired swallowing, altered bowel habit, loose-fitting clothes or prolonged intercurrent illness.

Malnourished:

BMI <18.5 kg/m^2
Unintentional weight loss >15% in 3–6 months
BMI <20 kg/m^2 and weight loss >5% in 3–6 months

At risk:

Poor absorptive capacity
Not eaten in five days; will not eat in next five days
High nutrient losses/requirements/catabolic

Ask:

Is patient safe to swallow? Do they have dysphagia?

If safe → oral feed

Malnourished/at risk → Inadequate/unsafe oral intake → a functional accessible GI tract → consider enteral tube feeding/post-pyloric feeding/ duodenal/jejunal feed

If >4 weeks feeding required consider percutaneous gastrostomy (PEG)

Can be used four hours after insertion.

Nasogastric tube (NGT) placement confirmation

NGT aspirate pH test <5.5 +/-Chest X-Ray (NPSA recommendation with senior doctor review of CXR)

Monitor for tube nasal erosion/blockage/fixation

Deliver enteral feed continuously over 16–24 hours. Four hourly NG aspirates in ICU.

If insulin infusion running → feed continuously or provide glucose intravenously to avoid hypoglycaemia.

Motility agents if delayed gastric emptying (e.g. metoclopramide iv 10 mg 8h ± erythromycin iv 200 mg 12h) – assess for high residual gastric volumes (>250–500 mL).

Consider post-pyloric feeding.

Maintaining gut transit time and avoiding constipation:

senna 10 mL daily (in all ICU patients on opioid infusions), then laxido sachet twice daily from 72 hours if persists. Rectal examination ± enema if persists thereafter.

Malnourished/at risk → Inadequate/unsafe oral intake → Non-functional/ leaking/perforated GI tract → Consider total parenteral nutrition (TPN)

Peripheral TPN if <14 days – pay attention to pH, tonicity and compatibility

If required for >30 days – will need tunnelled subclavian central venous catheter

Delivery – continuous. If required for >2 weeks, consider gradual change from continuous to cyclical.

TPN is introduced at <50% of needs over initial 24–48 hours.

Micronutrients and trace elements are added.

Stop when adequate enteral/oral intake.

SUMMARY OF NUTRITIONAL ASSESSMENT

Energy, protein, fluid, electrolyte, mineral, micronutrients and fibre needs
Activity levels and the underlying clinical condition
(catabolism, pyrexia, gastrointestinal tolerance, potential metabolic instability and risk of refeeding problems)
The likely duration of nutrition support.

REQUIREMENTS

NOT SEVERELY ILL OR INJURED PATIENTS WITHOUT RISK OF REFEEDING

Total energy 25–35 kcal/kg/day
Glucose 2 g/kg, Fat 2 g/kg, Protein 0.8–1.5 g/kg (0.13–0.24 g nitrogen/kg/day)
Water 30 mL/kg/day
or
100 mL/kg for 1st 10 kg; 50 mL/kg for next 10 kg; 20 mL/kg for each kg thereafter
per 24 hours
Sodium 1 mmol/kg/day
Potassium 1 mmol/kg/day
Magnesium and Calcium 0.1 mmol/kg/day
Phosphate 0.2 mmol/kg/day
Vitamins: C, A, D, E, K, Thiamine, Riboflavin, Niacin, Pyridoxine, Folate
Trace elements: Iron, Copper, Manganese, Zinc, Iodide, Fluoride

Example:

NG enteral isocalorific feeds, e.g. Osmolite©
Central TPN – Triomel N7 1140-E© at 40 mL/hr for 48 hours then increase to 55 mL/hr.
Peripheral TPN – Triomel N4 700E© at 60 mL/hr for 48 hours then increase to 90 mL/hr.

SERIOUSLY ILL OR INJURED PATIENTS

Introduce enteral or parenteral nutrition cautiously.

Start at no more than 50% of the estimated target energy and protein needs and build up to meet full needs over the first 48 hours. Provide full requirements of fluid, electrolytes, vitamins and minerals from the outset.

Calculation of energy requirements using the *Schofield* equation:

1. Calculate Basal Metabolic Rate (BMR) using: Admission weight(kg) × Factor + Factor (depends on age and gender; look up on tables)
2. Add stress factor, e.g. multiple trauma/severe sepsis + 30%
3. Add activity factor, e.g. bed bound + 10%, mobile + 25%
4. Reductions, e.g. on ventilator – 15%

Gives total kcal requirements per 24 hours

Nitrogen loss can be calculated to address the required intake but is notoriously inaccurate in critically ill patients:

24h nitrogen (g) loss = (urinary urea mmol·24h^{-1} × 0.028) + 4.0028

Approximately 4 g lost per day in faeces, skin, hair and urine as non-urea nitrogen.

REFEEDING SYNDROME

People who have eaten little or nothing for more than five days should have nutrition support introduced <50% of requirements for the first two days. In the absence of evidence of refeeding syndrome, increase feeding rates to meet full needs.

RISK FOR REFEEDING SYNDROME

One or more of the following:

- BMI less than 16 kg/m^2
- Unintentional weight loss greater than 15% within the last 3–6 months
- Little or no nutritional intake for more than 10 days
- Low levels of potassium, phosphate or magnesium prior to feeding

Two or more of the following:

- BMI less than 18.5 kg/m^2
- Unintentional weight loss >10% within 3–6 months
- Little or no nutritional intake for >5 days
- A history of alcohol abuse or drugs including insulin, chemotherapy, antacids or diuretics

PRESCRIPTION FOR PEOPLE AT HIGH RISK OF DEVELOPING REFEEDING PROBLEMS

Commence feed at maximum of 10 kcal/kg/day, increasing levels slowly to meet or exceed full needs by 4–7 days using only 5 kcal/kg/day.

Example:

Central TPN – Triomel N7 1140-E© at 20 mL/hr for 48 hours then increase to 30 mL/hr.

Peripheral TPN – Triomel N4 700E© at 30 mL/hr for 48 hours then increase to 50 mL/hr.

Intravenous vitamin B preparation (Pabrinex©) 'one pair' once daily for 10 days, 30 minutes prior to commencement of feed.

Balanced multivitamin/trace element supplement once daily.

Usual requirements in 'high risk for refeeding syndrome':

Potassium 2–4 mmol/kg/day
Phosphate 0.3–0.6 mmol/kg/day
Magnesium 0.2–0.4 mmol/kg/day

Monitor weight daily then weekly.

Body Mass Index (BMI)/triceps skin fold thickness/mid arm circumference at least monthly.

Monitoring nutrition in ICU:

Na, K, Urea, Creatinine, Mg, Ca, Albumin, LFTs, Glucose, Phosphate

Full Blood Count, Mean Cell Volume – looking for macrocytosis (MCV> 110 FL) associated with vitamin B12 and/or folate deficiency.

Serum folate/B12

Iron deficiency common with long-term parenteral feeding: Fe↓, Ferritin↑

If excessive fluid balance, 'double concentrate enteral feeds', e.g. TwoCal©, may be useful to maintain neutral fluid balance.

Rarely performed

Zinc, Copper deficiency – most at risk when anabolic

Selenium deficiency common after left hemicolectomy. Long-term status better assessed by glutathione peroxidase.

Avoid excessive manganese in liver disease (Red blood cell or whole blood better measure than serum)

1,25-dihydroxyvitamin D3 – requires working kidney

INTRAVENOUS FLUIDS

It is important to remember that fluid need not be administered intravenously and may be administered via the nasogastric tube as water.
Intravenous fluids:

Maintenance (0.18% sodium chloride (NaCl), 4% glucose with potassium chloride (KCl) 10–20 mmol/L depending on plasma potassium level) at 1 mL/kg/hr.

Replacement/resuscitative losses (e.g. blood, gastrointestinal fluid, sweating) 'balanced' crystalloid solutions (PlasmaLyte 148, Compound Sodium Lactate or Hartmann's).

'Normal saline' (0.9% NaCl) contains excessive sodium and chloride (154 mmol/L) compared to body plasma and may cause hyperchloraemic acidosis. However, it can be appropriate, for e.g. gastric outlet obstruction.

Dextrose-containing solutions have the advantage of providing glucose but are hypotonic and are rapidly distributed beyond the extracellular fluid space.

Colloids (salt-balanced gelatins and human albumin solutions) are generally reserved for resuscitation of the intravascular compartment in hypotension if adequate crystalloid resuscitation has failed. There is no clinical outcome benefit of colloids over crystalloids though albumin may have a role in early severe sepsis.

FURTHER READING

Casaer, Michael P., Dieter Mesotten, Greet Hermans, Pieter J. Wouters, Miet Schetz, Geert Meyfroidt, Sophie van Cromphaut, Catherine Ingels,

Philippe Meersseman, Jan Muller, Dirk Vlasselaers, Yves Debaveye, Lars Desmet, Jasperina Dubois, Aime van Assche, Simon Vanderheyden, Alexander Wilmer, and Greet van den Berghe. "Early versus Late Parenteral Nutrition in Critically Ill Adults." *New England Journal of Medicine* 365, no. 6 (August 2011): 506–517.

Doig, Gordon S., Fiona Simpson, Elizabeth A. Sweetman, Simon R. Finfer, D. Jamie Cooper, Philippa T. Heighes, Andrew R. Davies, Michael O'Leary, Tom Solano, Sandra Peake, for the Early PN Investigators of the ANZICS Clinical Trials Group. "Early Parenteral Nutrition in Critically Ill Patients with Short-Term Relative Contraindications to Early Enteral Nutrition: A Randomized Controlled Trial." *Journal of the American Medical Association* 309, no. 20 (2013): 2130–2138.

National Heart, Lung, and Blood Institute Acute Respiratory Distress Syndrome (ARDS) Clinical Trials Network. "Initial Trophic vs Full Enteral Feeding in Patients with Acute Lung Injury: The EDEN Randomized Trial." *Journal of the American Medical Association* 307, no. 8 (2012): 795–803.

National Institute for Health and Care Excellence. "Nutrition Support in Adults." Quality standard QS24, National Institute for Health and Care Excellence, Manchester, UK, November 2012 (updated March 2017).

National Institute for Health and Care Excellence. "Intravenous Fluid Therapy in Adults in Hospital." Clinical guideline CG174, National Institute for Health and Care Excellence, Manchester, UK, December 2013 (updated May 2017).

Powell-Tuck, Jeremy, Peter Gosling, Dileep N. Lobo, Simon P. Allison, Gordon L. Carlson, Marcus Gore, Andrew J. Lewington, Rupert M. Pearse, and Monty G. Mythen. "British Consensus Guidelines on Intravenous Fluid Therapy for Adult Surgical Patients: GIFTASUP." www.bapen.org.uk/pdfs/bapen_pubs/giftasup.pdf.

Preiser, Jean-Charles, Arthur R.H. van Zanten, Mette M. Berger, Gianni Biolo, Michael P. Casaer, Gordon S. Doig, Richard D. Griffiths, Daren K. Heyland, Michael Hiesmayr, Gaetano Iapichino, Alessandro Laviano, Claude Pichard, Pierre Singer, Greet van den Berghe, Jan Wernerman, Paul Wischmeyer, and Jean-Louis Vincent. "Metabolic and Nutritional Support of Critically Ill Patients: Consensus and Controversies." *Critical Care* 19, no. 1 (2015): 35.

PART 5

EQUIPMENT AND INVESTIGATIONS

20

Face masks, continuous positive airway pressure (CPAP) and airways

ANNA HERBERT AND SHONDIPON K. LAHA

'How much oxygen do you want for this patient?'

You are asked to review a 70-year-old gentleman on the acute medical unit (AMU) who has been admitted with CURB 3 community-acquired pneumonia. His oxygen requirements have increased over the past four hours since admission from 2 L O_2 via nasal cannula to 10 L O_2 via simple face mask.

He is feeling short of breath, with a respiratory rate of 28 breaths/min and SpO$_2$ 90%. His ABG shows a pH of 7.37, pO$_2$ 9.0 and PaCO$_2$ 4.79, with a normal metabolic profile. He has no significant cardiorespiratory past medical history, a good exercise tolerance when well and is a lifelong non-smoker. The medical team are concerned that his oxygen requirements are rapidly increasing and are reaching the ceiling of care available on a medical ward.

They plan to increase his oxygen supply to 15 L O_2 via a non-rebreathe mask and have requested your input into his care.

LEARNING OBJECTIVES

- Understand the advantages and disadvantages of various methods of oxygen delivery, and the main differences between them.
- Start to think about higher levels of respiratory support, including methods of securing the airway.
- Consider the clinical scenario and formulate a management plan, taking into account the need for oxygen delivery and any respiratory support required.

INTRODUCTION

Basic assessment and resuscitation of any critically ill patient follow an ABCDE approach:

- **A**irway
- **B**reathing
- **C**irculation
- **D**isability
- **E**xposure

Effective ventilation requires a patent airway, movement of oxygen and carbon dioxide in and out of the airways into the lungs and gas exchange between the alveoli and pulmonary circulation. This is the ultimate aim of **A**irway and **B**reathing.

In this chapter, we will discuss the various methods of effectively managing and supporting the airway and breathing in critical care, including their merits and limitations. Some of these methods will be familiar to you and are commonplace in any acute inpatient ward. However, some methods can only be safely delivered and monitored in a level 2 or 3 environment. The choice of oxygen delivery device will depend upon the amount of oxygen required, additional respiratory support needed and patient compliance.

OXYGEN DELIVERY WITHOUT AIRWAY OR RESPIRATORY SUPPORT

Your ABCDE assessment of the patient has identified that the patient is hypoxic, but maintaining their own airway, breathing spontaneously and not demonstrating any features of respiratory distress. In this situation, supplemental oxygen is all that is required in the first instance. Depending on the percentage of oxygen that you wish to deliver, there is a choice of devices available.

The amount of oxygen that is being provided is expressed as a percentage (%) or fraction of inspired oxygen (FiO_2), with 100% O_2 being equivalent to an FiO_2 of 1.0. Flow rates are expressed in litres per minute (L/min). Room air delivers 21% oxygen (FiO_2 0.21).

NASAL CANNULAE

These are clear prongs that fit into each nostril, with tubing secured behind the ears and under the chin. They can deliver between 24%–35% oxygen with flow rates of 2–4 L/min. A higher FiO_2 can be achieved with flow rates up to 6 L/min if tolerated. The advantages and disadvantages of nasal cannulae are summarised below:

Advantages	Disadvantages
• Minimally disruptive and well tolerated within limitations of flow rate • The patient can eat, drink and talk normally	• Only air entered through the nose is supplemented with oxygen • Higher flow rates can cause discomfort and bleeding • Cannot reliably determine how much oxygen the patient is receiving • Only suitable for patients with lower oxygen requirements

SIMPLE (HUDSON) FACE MASK

Air is mixed with oxygen within a clear mask that fits around the mouth and nose, and breathed in by the patient. A minimum of 5 L/min oxygen flow is required to ensure expired carbon dioxide is removed from the mask chamber, and not rebreathed. With flow rates of 5–10 L/min, it can deliver between 35% and 60% oxygen. However, with air and oxygen being mixed in varying ratios, it is not possible to determine exactly how much oxygen is being inspired.

This form of oxygen delivery is more disrupting to the patient. The mask requires removal to eat and drink and the higher flow rates can rapidly dry out the upper airways, potentially reducing its tolerance. If this level of supplemental oxygen is expected to be required for a prolonged period of time, humidified oxygen delivery should be considered. This will keep the airways and any secretions moist, facilitating expectoration and becoming potentially more tolerable to the patient.

VENTURI FACE MASK

These masks are used to deliver a fixed percentage of oxygen – the only method available to do so via a simple face mask. A Venturi mask consists of a face mask attached to a valve that will entrain a fixed amount of oxygen through the valve. At a set flow rate, this air and oxygen mix will deliver a specific percentage of oxygen into the mask for inspiration.

There are five different valves available, each colour-coded with a specified oxygen flow rate in L/min and the percentage of oxygen that the given flow rate will deliver written on the side of the mask. The percentages available are 24%, 28%, 35%, 40% and 60% oxygen.

You may have seen these masks used where controlled oxygen therapy is required, typically in COPD patients, where the level of hypoxia to be corrected has to be carefully balanced against their respiratory (hypoxic) drive.

FACE MASK WITH RESERVOIR BAG

Also known as a non-rebreathe mask, this is a clear mask with a one-way valve and a reservoir bag beneath it. Once the reservoir bag is inflated, 100% oxygen contained within the bag is inspired through the one-way valve. As this oxygen passes through the face mask into the patient, it will inevitably mix with room air and expired carbon dioxide contained within the mask.

However, it still provides 80%–98% inspired oxygen when provided with a flow rate of 15 L/min and is the highest oxygen-delivery method of all the supplemental oxygen devices listed above.

Once any of these methods of oxygen delivery have been administered, remember to reassess your patient using the ABCDE approach, ensuring the method chosen is sufficient for the patient's needs. A regular re-review is required to escalate or de-escalate the oxygen therapy as needed.

OXYGEN DELIVERY WITH RESPIRATORY SUPPORT

Your ABCDE assessment may indicate that the patient requires more than just supplemental oxygen in supporting breathing, particularly if the following features are present:

1. The need for high-flow oxygen therapy (FiO_2 of 60% or more), titrated against the target SpO_2 or PaO_2 on the ABG.
2. A type 2 respiratory failure on the ABG (acutely elevated CO_2 with acidosis).
3. Evidence of respiratory distress – dyspnoeic and tachypnoeic, use of accessory muscles of respiration, unable to complete full sentences in one breath.

In these situations, extra-respiratory support is likely to be required. First, you need to decide if the patient requires respiratory support in the form of continuous positive airway pressure (CPAP), providing positive end-expiratory pressure (PEEP), or if they require ventilatory support in the form of non-invasive positive pressure ventilation (NIPPV), also referred to as BiPAP (bi-level positive airway pressure) or NIV (non-invasive ventilation).

The distinction between respiratory and ventilatory support is important, as it ensures the correct method of support if chosen in the correct circumstance.

HIGH-FLOW NASAL CANNULA (HFNC)

This form of oxygen therapy consists of wide-bore nasal cannulae attached to an air–oxygen mixer, providing heated and humidified oxygen up to 70 L/min flow. The flow of oxygen is much greater than the 15 L/min, which can be provided via standard face masks, and is substantially greater than that which can be provided via conventional nasal cannulae due to much wider tubing. This high flow rate can deliver PEEP up to 3 cmH_2O. The PEEP prevents alveolar collapse at the end of expiration, facilitating greater gas exchange within the alveolae and reducing the work of breathing required to keep these alveolae open. In conjunction with a fixed percentage oxygen delivery up to FiO_2 70%, HFNC can be used to improve oxygenation and reduce work of breathing.

Much like the standard nasal cannulae, HFNC has the advantage of being less disruptive than face masks and generally well tolerated compared to other forms of respiratory support.

However, whilst the percentage oxygen and flow rate can be altered, the amount of PEEP generated cannot be measured and for patients who require greater PEEP for respiratory support, escalation to CPAP may be required.

CONTINUOUS POSITIVE AIRWAY PRESSURE (CPAP)

CPAP can be delivered either via a tight-fitting mask that is strapped around the head, and fits over the mouth and nose or via a hood that encloses the entire head and fits tightly around the neck. It is possible to alter the PEEP, oxygen percentage and oxygen flow rate. CPAP aims to improve oxygenation and reduce work of breathing. The continuous airway pressure will provide a peak end expiratory pressure (PEEP) that prevents alveolar collapse at the end of expiration, facilitating greater gas exchange within the alveolae and reducing the work of breathing required to keep these alveolae open.

As with HFNC, the flow of oxygen delivered can be much greater than the rate of 15 L/min due to sider tubing, improving overall oxygenation, but with the additional benefit of a greater, measurable and titratable PEEP.

However, CPAP can be claustrophobic and the sensation of the continuous positive pressure can be difficult to tolerate. The mask requires removal or the hood deflating via a side window to allow the patient to eat and drink. In these circumstances, it can be useful to temporarily de-escalate the respiratory support to HFNC, preventing all support provided by the CPAP from being lost.

NON-INVASIVE POSITIVE PRESSURE VENTILATION (NIPPV/BIPAP/NIV)

This uses the same tight-fitting mask as with CPAP. NIPPV provides ventilatory support, as both inspiration and expiration are supported via two alternating levels of pressure, both of which can be separately adjusted. The higher pressure provides inspiratory pressure support, to reduce the work of breathing during inspiration, and the lower pressure provides the PEEP, preventing alveolar collapse with expiration. The inspiratory pressure effectively forces air into the patient's lungs as they breathe in, and this sensation may not be tolerated by some patients, often to a greater extent than with CPAP.

NIPPV can be used for a number of reasons, but is particularly efficacious in patients with type 2 respiratory failure, for the purpose of both improving oxygenation and carbon dioxide reduction, and in patients who require ventilatory support but might not be suitable for invasive ventilation.

For all forms of non-invasive respiratory support, there should be a well documented plan regarding the management steps if it should fail to improve the patient's breathing, and whether progression to invasive ventilation would be suitable. Ideally, this should be discussed with the patient prior to commencement of respiratory support, and their wishes should be sorted to guide decision making where appropriate.

OXYGEN DELIVERING WITH AIRWAY SUPPORT

This section introduces the two most common forms of airway support in the critical care setting; an endotracheal tube (ETT) and a tracheostomy. These devices are adjuncts to secure a patent airway in a patient who requires invasive ventilation or who has a low Glasgow Coma Scale (GCS) and is unable to protect their airway independently as a consequence. These devices are positioned in the airway to keep it patent and can be attached to a ventilator or CPAP machine to provide both airway and respiratory support.

ENDOTRACHEAL TUBE (ETT)

An ETT is a clear flexible tube with length markings (in cm) along the side and a surrounding inflatable cuff at the distal end. It is inserted through the mouth, past the vocal cords and into the trachea, viewed via a laryngoscope, while the patient is sedated. The cuff is then inflated from a port at the proximal end to occlude the airway around the tube. The tube is secured in place with either tape or a mask attached to the tube and fitted to the face. If this insertion method proves difficult, there are other advanced techniques that are not covered in this chapter. The insertion of an ETT should always be performed by a skilled airway-trained practitioner.

ETTs are available in a range of diameters, but typically size 7.0 for females and size 8.0 for males is used.

The main risks associated with the use of an ETT are increased risk of pneumonia, due to the inability of the patient to occlude the vocal cords, creating an open passage from the outside air directly to the lungs, and pooling of secretions of the inflated cuff, which can trickle down into the lungs, leading to infection.

The inflated cuff can cause tracheal stenosis if it is too inflated or sited for too long. If longer-term support is needed, a tracheostomy may be required.

TRACHEOSTOMY

A tracheostomy is inserted when a patient is likely to require longer-term airway support. A tracheostomy is a curved tube with an inflatable cuff that sits in the trachea, below the vocal cords and is secured by tape strapped around the neck. As with an ET tube, both mechanical ventilation and spontaneous breathing are possible via a tracheostomy, including CPAP.

Tracheostomy insertion can be performed percutaneously on the critical care unit, or surgically in theatre. Anticipated complications due to patient anatomy and bleeding risk are often the deciding factors as to which method is preferred.

As the tracheostomy does not pass through the vocal cords, it can be fitted with a speaking (or Passy Muir) valve. When the cuff surrounding the tracheostomy is deflated, this one-way valve allows the patient to breathe in through the tube and out past the tracheostomy and vocal cords through their nose and mouth, generating speech as they do so.

CLINICAL SCENARIO MANAGEMENT PLAN

Hopefully you are now better equipped to manage the clinical scenario at the beginning of the chapter. In this scenario, it is clear that the patient's respiratory function is acutely worsening. He is dyspnoeic and tachypnoeic, with evidence of respiratory distress. His oxygen requirements have increased over a short period of time, with low peripheral saturations and a type 1 respiratory failure demonstrated on the ABG. The medical team are planning to increase his oxygen delivery further with the use of a non-rebreathe mask and 15 L/min oxygen flow, but it would appear that this man needs additional respiratory support. In the first instance, it would be reasonable to trial HFNC, but given the high oxygen requirements and current work of breathing, this may be insufficient and escalation to CPAP or even invasive ventilation with a secure airway may be required.

Advice from senior clinicians in both critical care and the patient's medical team should be used in making these decisions, and an escalation plan should be formulated and discussed with the patient prior to intervention if possible.

The ventilator

IRFAN CHAUDRY

'What settings do you want on the ventilator for this patient, doctor?'

We will look at the very basics around why we ventilate a patient and the settings used. A basic knowledge of respiratory physiology and respiratory failure will be assumed for this chapter. This will focus on the use of invasive ventilation. More advanced methods of ventilating patients are outside the scope of this chapter and readers are directed to the further reading section.

LEARNING OBJECTIVES

- Why do we need to ventilate?
- How to set up the ventilator.
- Common pitfalls and complications.

WHY DO WE NEED TO VENTILATE?

We need to ventilate patients for various reasons. These can be split broadly into two categories.

Extra-pulmonary

CENTRAL NERVOUS SYSTEM

- Coma
- Overdose on sedative or narcotic medication
- Failure of respiratory centres

NEUROMUSCULAR

- Myasthenia gravis
- Electrolyte imbalance
- Diaphragmatic dysfunction

MUSCULOSKELETAL

- Trauma
- Flail chest

Pulmonary

- Airway obstruction
- Non-compliant lung tissue, e.g. pneumonia, ARDS

For the reasons listed above, we need to augment normal respiratory function and this basically means getting oxygen from the atmosphere into the tissues and removing carbon dioxide from the tissues via the lungs causing minimal damage on the way!

We will assume that the patient has been connected to the ventilator via a closed suction device and some form of humidification.

Most modern ICUs use positive pressure to drive air/oxygen into patients' lungs through an interface, which may be an endotracheal tube or a tracheostomy. Hence, this is known as IPPV (Intermittent Positive Pressure Ventilation). Non-invasive ventilation uses a face mask or hood, and has different terminology. The basics of ventilation, however, remain similar.

HOW TO SET UP THE VENTILATOR

The first aim of ventilation is getting oxygen into the patient:

- *PaO$_2$*: by altering the inspired oxygen concentration (**FiO$_2$**), the alveolar pressure and alveolar ventilation
- *Ventilation/Perfusion (V/Q) ratio*: by recruiting collapsed alveoli to reduce the amount of intra pulmonary shunt; this can be done using **PEEP** (Positive end-expiratory pressure), usually 5–10 cmH$_2$O

The second aim is to get carbon dioxide out of the patient – manipulating alveolar ventilation does this:

- *Alveolar ventilation* = Respiratory rate × (Tidal volume – dead space volume)

The third aim is to minimise any damage caused to the pulmonary system:

- *Volutrauma:* damage due to volume overload of the alveoli
- *Barotrauma:* damage due to pressure overload of the alveoli

Aim for tidal volumes of 6–8 mL/kg in non-compliant lungs (up to 10 mL/kg in 'normal' lungs) and, mean airway pressures of around 25–30 cmH$_2$O. Peak pressures greater than 45 cmH$_2$O or plateau pressures >30 cmH$_2$O are associated with alveolar damage (see Chapter 40 on ARDS).

The mode of ventilation is also important when setting up:

CMV: Continuous mandatory ventilation, i.e. all respiratory movements are made by the ventilator with no patient input. Very few patients will be on this mode.

SIMV: Synchronised intermittent mandatory ventilation, i.e. the patient has respiratory effort and this is synchronised with ventilator-delivered breaths. The mandatory breaths can be volume-controlled (traditional) or pressure-controlled (PSIMV). The ventilator generally supports patient-initiated breaths with pressure support.

SPONT: This is a spontaneous mode where the patient initiates breaths on his or her own, usually with some form of support, e.g. pressure support.

There are special modes like Airway Pressure Release Ventilation (APRV).

Different manufacturers may have different names for these modes in their ventilators. For instance, spontaneous mode may be called Pressure Support or Assisted Spontaneous Breathing (ASB).

Next, decide on whether ventilator breaths are to be volume controlled (VCV) or pressure controlled (PCV).

So as an example, a starting point for a 70-kg man could be

- FiO_2 100%
- SIMV, VCV tidal volume set at 500 mL, rate set at 12 breaths/min
- PEEP 5 cmH_2O

Remember to use measured parameters (e.g. SaO_2 or arterial blood gases) and clinical assessment (e.g. is the patient synchronising with the ventilator to guide further settings?).

Common adjustments you may have to make would be

1. Patient has low PaO_2: this can be remedied by increasing the FiO_2 or increasing PEEP if you think the problem is de-recruitment.
2. Patient has high $PaCO_2$: The patient needs an increase in minute volume. This may be achieved by either increasing the rate or increasing the tidal volume (making sure you stay in safe limits).

COMMON PITFALLS AND COMPLICATIONS

As with all problems with ventilated patients, check your patient first before checking the ventilator. If the problem is with the ventilator, remember you can isolate the patient by manual ventilation with a resuscitation bag.

- *Ventilator-associated lung injury*: this can be avoided by using lung protective strategies (see Chapter 40 on ARDS).
- *Barotrauma*, e.g. pneumothorax or air embolism: this can be avoided by not using excess pressures.
- *Cardiovascular compromise* due to excessive intra-thoracic pressure and poor venous return: again, avoid excess pressure and PEEP.
- *Raised intracranial pressures*: again could be due to increased intra-thoracic pressure or raised $PaCO_2$ (see Chapter 15 on head injuries).
- *Ventilator-associated pneumonia*: adopting an appropriate package of care may reduce the risk.

WEANING

This is actually the process of liberating the patient from mechanical ventilation. Weaning must not be ignored when a patient is ventilated.

Generally, successful weaning needs the patient's underlying health condition, which caused them to be ventilated, to start getting better. The patient also needs to be calm, neurologically intact and to have adequate strength.

Sedation holds, lung-protective ventilation and daily spontaneous breathing have been shown to improve weaning.

Weaning may be accomplished by

1. Moving patients to less dependent forms of ventilation, e.g. moving from CMV to SIMV and then spontaneous mode
2. Decreasing the pressure support gradually
3. Periods of CPAP/spontaneous breathing trials with minimal or no pressure support

Generally a mix of these strategies is used in most units.

Some patients may wean slowly and need weaning plans that are tailored to them.

KEY LEARNING POINTS

- There are pulmonary and non-pulmonary reasons for requiring mechanical ventilation.
- The three aims of ventilation are to get oxygen in, carbon dioxide out and minimise pulmonary trauma.
- Invasive ventilation can have significant complications.
- Weaning is important and must start early.

FURTHER READING

The Acute Respiratory Distress Syndrome Network. "Ventilation with Lower Tidal Volumes as Compared with Traditional Tidal Volumes for Acute Lung Injury and the Acute Respiratory Distress Syndrome." *New England Journal of Medicine* 342, no. 18 (May 2000): 1301–1308.

Bersten, Andrew, and Neil Soni. *Oh's Intensive Care Manual,* 6th ed. Philadelphia: Butterworth Heinemann (Elsevier), 2009.

Whitehead, Tom, and Arthur S. Slutsky. "The Pulmonary Physician in Critical Care 7: Ventilator Induced Lung Injury." *Thorax* 57 (2002): 635–642.

22

Monitoring the critical care patient

ROCHELLE VELHO AND ROBERT O'BRIEN

*'Mrs Moffat in Bed 3 is four days post-oesophagostomy. She has spiked a tem-
perature of 39.1°C, and her heart rate is elevated at 128 bpm. Please can you
come and review her?'*

A clinical review of an intensive care patient happens periodically at
planned ward rounds and unplanned time points throughout a clinical shift.
These reviews integrate the history, examination findings and the trend in
physiological parameters to help clinicians optimise the patient's management plan.

As a novice to the critical care setting, it can be daunting to be faced by
all the measuring devices attached to the patients, especially when they trigger an alarm. Daily patient observations are recorded to help the intensive
care unit (ICU) team identify the trend in common physiological parameters,
which are associated with changes in different body systems. Although different ICUs use different measuring devices, the combination of recorded
monitoring values is likely to be the same. The standards for monitoring are
outlined by different professional bodies for the ICU environment and for
transfer of the ICU patient (Checketts, 2015; Interhospital Transfer, 2009;
NICE Guideline, 2017). In the ICU setting, monitoring should be used as an
adjunct and not as a replacement for clinical assessment.

The key parameters used to monitor an ICU patient can be categorised
using the ABC framework and are outlined as follows.

AIRWAY

END TIDAL CAPNOMETRY ($ETCO_2$)

This is usually presented as a capnograph and a number. It monitors the
concentration or partial pressure of carbon dioxide (CO_2) in the respiratory
gases. You can also check the oxygen delivery, tube cuff pressure and ascertain whether there is a leak. A normal range is 4–5.7 kPa.

BREATHING

RESPIRATORY RATE

This is measured via the ECG electrodes or counted manually. The normal range for adults is 12–20 breaths per minute.

OXYGEN SATURATION

This is measured using a pulse oximeter and gives an indication of oxygenation not ventilation. If the patient is peripherally shut down, earlobe probes may give a more accurate reading. For adults without pre-existing lung pathology, the normal range for oxygen saturation is 98 to 100 per cent.

VENTILATOR VALUES

Check the ventilator settings, but essentially is this patient on the right ventilator settings to deliver oxygen and extract carbon dioxide from the lungs? Take paralysis into account and level of consciousness. Escalate if necessary.

ARTERIAL BLOOD GAS

This will enable you to elicit whether there is a respiratory or metabolic issue.

CIRCULATION

HEART RATE

Heart rate can be measured by the ECG electrodes, pulse oximeter or manually. The normal range for adults is 60–100 beats per minute. Less than 60 indicates bradycardia; more than 100 indicates tachycardia.

ELECTROCARDIOGRAM (ECG)

This trace is a representation on a monitor of the electrical activity of the heart. If the trace appears abnormal, it is worth checking the arterial line trace (if available) for concordant abnormal activity. Normal and abnormal ECG traces are beyond the scope of this chapter.

BLOOD PRESSURE AND MEAN ARTERIAL BLOOD PRESSURE (MAP)

The target is to maintain adequate perfusion to the vital organs (e.g. urine output as a marker of kidney perfusion) and its 'normal values' are individualised to the patient. This can be measured non-invasively or invasively. Non-invasive blood pressure can be measured using a cuff on either the upper or lower limb.

Invasive blood pressure can be achieved using an arterial line. Arterial lines are sited in an artery (usually radial, but femoral, brachial and dorsalis pedis may be used) connected to a transducer that generates a continuous blood pressure trace. This line also enables regular blood sampling through arterial lines.

MAP is defined as the average pressure over a whole cardiac cycle and can be deduced from the systolic and diastolic values. The MAP is usually displayed in brackets after the BP.

CENTRAL LINES AND CENTRAL VENOUS PRESSURE (CVP)

These are catheters that are fed into the large 'central' vein (femoral, internal jugular or subclavian) and again connected to a transducer. They give a measurement of venous blood pressure and allow administration of total parenteral nutrition, medication and fluid into a large vein. This could also be required if medication cannot be administered peripherally or if venous access is particularly difficult. In the majority of patients, central venous pressure can be used as a reflection of right (and thus left) ventricular preload. The exceptions to this are patients with severe ventricular dysfunction, pulmonary hypertension and those on mechanical ventilation. The range of normal CVP values is 3–8 mmHg.

CARDIAC OUTPUT MONITORING

This includes oesophageal Doppler monitoring (ODM), pulse contour cardiac output monitoring (PiCCO) and lithium dilution cardiac output monitoring (LiDCO). ODM measures the blood flow velocity in the descending aorta using a flexible ultrasound probe and the Doppler principle. The PiCCO and LiDCO monitors both analyse peripheral arterial waveforms but are calibrated using different methods. The PiCCO method uses transpulmonary thermodilution to measure temperatures changes from a central venous line to a central arterial line as the calibrating technique. Whilst the older LiDCO method uses lithium chloride dilution to calibrate, the newer LiDCOrapid monitor makes use of a nomogram-based estimate according to patient age, height and weight to calibrate the arterial waveform. All these techniques estimate the cardiac output, stroke volume and systemic vascular resistance that aid goal directed therapy in ICU patients to optimise cardiovascular function.

ECHOCARDIOGRAM

Please see Chapter 23 about ultrasound in ICU.

DISABILITY

GLASGOW COMA SCALE (GCS)

This is a neurological scale to objectively determine the conscious level of a patient that is not tubed. In the tubed patient, a sedation score can be employed. Three components of the GCS evaluate eyes, motor and verbal response. A normal GCS ranges from 3 to 15.

CAPILLARY BLOOD GLUCOSE

This is an important measure and may be obtained from the arterial line or a finger prick. This is individualised and also depends on whether the patient has diabetes mellitus. For a fasting adult ICU patient, a normal range is 3.9–5.5 mmol/L.

INTRACRANIAL PRESSURE (ICP)

This is a measurement of pressure inside the cranial vault. It is measured via an ICP bolt connected to a transducer. Raised ICP is quite common when weaning patients off sedation.

EXPOSURE

TEMPERATURE

This will usually be recorded using a tympanic thermometer. A normal range is 36.5–37.2 degrees Celsius.

URINE OUTPUT

The majority of patients will be catheterised to measure hourly urine output. This can then be compared to fluid input over the same period, to assess overall fluid balance. A normal value is greater than 1 mL/kg/hr.

There are other more specialist monitors that you may come across in the critical care setting, such as BIS monitoring, to be aware of but which are not detailed here.

WHICH OF THESE PARAMETERS ARE IMPORTANT FOR YOUR CLINICAL REVIEW OF MRS MOFFAT?

Remember to go back to basics and use a systematic ABC approach, as it can be distracting to focus only on the monitoring and the alarms.

As a junior doctor, ask yourself: is this an emergency? Follow ALS algorithms and escalate early. In this case, start by gaining more information and looking at the history; the SBAR framework can help clarify the case. You find that the patient has been on ICU for four days and spiked a temperature last night as well. Cultures were sent but are not back yet, and the patient is on broad-spectrum antibiotics as per a microbiology review.

Starting with an airway assessment in an intubated patient like Mrs Moffat, and check the tube. Is it displaced, are there secretions obstructing it or is there an equipment malfunction? The $ETCO_2$ was 5 in this patient so you proceed to your next step. On chest examination, there are coarse crackles on the right base and there are thick secretions from the ETT. The saturations are 92% with an FiO_2 of 0.4. With regard to circulation, the patient is in sinus tachycardia when you see her at 132 bpm, with a MAP of 60 and this has been a persistent tachycardia for the last 30 minutes. She is having a unit of blood that started 20 minutes ago for a low haemoglobin (72 g/L). The patient is sedated and has a sedation score of –2, the capillary blood glucose is 5.5, and the pupils are equal and reacting. On exposure, you see an urticarial rash on her legs and hands with no associated angioedema.

Your main differential diagnosis is an allergic reaction to a blood product, so what will your management plan be? Stop the blood transfusion and then treat the allergic reaction as per protocol. However, it is never straightforward. Mrs Moffat may also have a chest sepsis and the rash may be due to an infection. Remember to escalate to your senior as soon as possible.

The main learning point is that monitoring does not replace clinical history and examination, but is an invaluable adjunct to diagnose and manage an ICU patient.

FURTHER READING

Association of Anaesthetists of Great Britain and Ireland. "Interhospital Transfer." AAGBI Safety Guideline, The Association of Anaesthetists of Great Britain and Ireland, London, February 2009.

Checketts, M.R., R. Alladi, K. Ferguson, L. Gemmell, J. M. Handy, A. A. Klein, N. J. Love, U. Misra, C. Morris, M. H. Nathanson, G. E. Rodney, R. Verma, and J. J. Pandit. "Recommendations for Standards of Monitoring during Anaesthesia and Recovery 2015: The Association of Anaesthetists of Great Britain and Ireland." *Anaesthesia* 71, no. 1 (January 2016): 85–93.

National Institute for Health and Care Excellence. "Acutely Ill Adults in Hospital: Recognising and Responding to Deterioration." Clinical guideline CG50, National Institute for Health and Care Excellence, Manchester, UK, July 2007 (updated March 2016).

23

Ultrasound in intensive care

ADRIAN WONG AND OLUSEGUN OLUSANYA

Mark, who is normally fit and well, has just been admitted to the emergency department after being increasingly feverish and lethargic for the last four days. He is found to be hypoxic, hypotensive and oliguric by the Emergency Department (ED) team. How would you diagnose and guide therapy in this situation?

Patients who present themselves in multi-organ failure to the ED require prompt diagnosis and management. The use of point-of-care ultrasound scans allows for the rapid assessment and diagnosis of conditions immediately by the bedside without the use of ionising radiation. Ultrasound as an imaging modality has evolved beyond the remit of the radiologist into a powerful tool of the intensive care physician.

WHAT IS ULTRASOUND?

Medical ultrasound involves the use of high frequency sound waves (beyond the audible range) to create an image of the various parts of the body. The sound waves are created by passing an electrical current across a special (piezoelectric) crystal. As they travel through the area of interest, the waves are reflected by the various organs and tissue to a varying extent. The reflected waves are detected by the same crystals to generate an image.

HOW CAN ULTRASOUND HELP IN INTENSIVE CARE?

Once used purely as a diagnostic tool by the radiologist, its role has expanded into all areas of medicine including the acute specialties such as intensive care. Beyond answering clinical questions, it also has a role in monitoring, therapeutic and aiding invasive procedures.

There is no limit to the various modalities or organs that can be imaged with ultrasound and its use continues to expand. The most common modalities in the intensive care setting are

- Echocardiography
- Lung ultrasound
- Abdominal ultrasound
- Vascular ultrasound

As technology improves, the miniaturisation of the ultrasound machine continues. The use of hand-held ultrasound devices allows for rapid assessment of the patient by the bedside.

ECHOCARDIOGRAPHY

Echocardiography can be divided into trans-thoracic or trans-oesophageal. By far the most accessible (and which will be discussed here) is trans-thoracic. A focused echocardiographic examination allows for an assessment of

- Left ventricular size and function
- Right ventricular size and function

- Presence/absence of pericardial effusion and tamponade
- Valvular function
- IVC size and dynamics

Putting all of these components together means that the various subtypes of shock can be differentiated and diagnosed. An accurate diagnosis means that treatment strategies can be put in place and efficacy monitored. Furthermore, the patients' fluid status and response to fluid therapy can be assessed and monitored.

There are several standard views for trans-thoracic echocardiography:

- Parasternal long axis (PLAX) (Figure 23.1)
- Parasternal short axis (PSAX) (Figure 23.2)
- Apical 4 Chamber (Figure 23.3)
- Subcostal (Figure 23.4)

The three other views (two-chamber, three-chamber, and suprasternal) are not commonly used in the intensive care population.

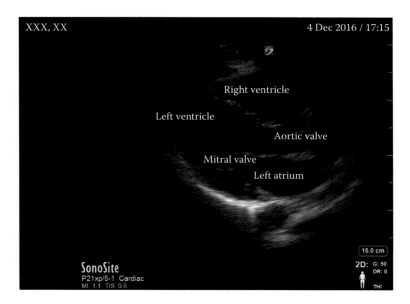

Figure 23.1 Parasternal long axis view.

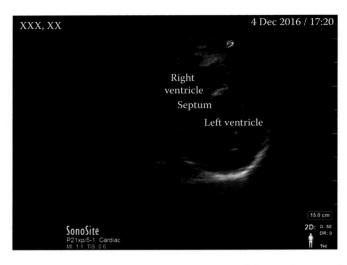

Figure 23.2 Parasternal short axis view at the level of the papillary muscles.

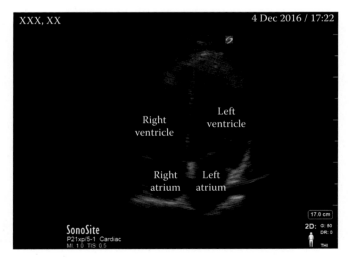

Figure 23.3 Apical 4 Chamber view.

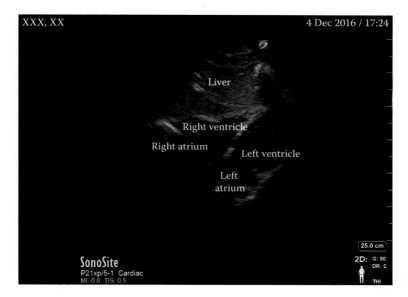

Figure 23.4 Subcostal long axis view.

LUNG ULTRASOUND

The use of lung ultrasound in the ICU began as an aid to drain pleural effusions. Traditionally, failure to tap an effusion using landmark/clinical examination led to a phone call to the radiologist to help mark an insertion point using ultrasound. This practice has now evolved into real-time guidance where ultrasound is used to visualise the needle puncture and the pleural cavity (Figure 23.5).

More recently, the use of ultrasound as a tool in the diagnosis of lung pathology has expanded. Whilst the normal lung is relatively unexciting when visualised with an ultrasound probe, its appearance changes when there is disease. These changes can then be used in a stepwise diagnostic template, such as the BLUE and SESAME protocol. There is increasing evidence that ultrasound is superior to clinical examination and plain chest radiographs in diagnosing a range of pathologies (Figure 23.6).

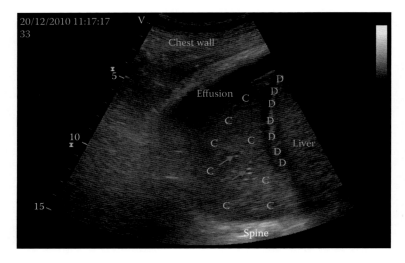

Figure 23.5 Right lower zone lung ultrasound showing consolidated lung (C) with surrounding effusion, seen as the dark hypoechoic zone around it. Air bronchograms also noted (arrows). D = diaphragm.

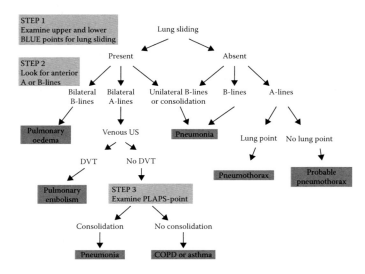

Figure 23.6 BLUE protocol for lung ultrasound.

ABDOMINAL ULTRASOUND

The potential uses of ultrasound in the abdomen as both a diagnostic tool and to aid interventional procedures is vast. As an aid to intervention, like aspiration of pleural effusions, real-time ultrasound to drain ascitic fluid is clearly safer for patients. Indeed, drainage of other collections visualised by ultrasound, e.g. liver abscesses, gallbladder empyemas, and perinephric fluid, are made possible and safer through the use of ultrasound. Ultrasound can also be used for suprapubic catheterisation, and for visual confirmation of urethral catheterisation and nasogastric tube insertion.

Most major viscera – the stomach, liver, spleen, pancreas, gallbladder, small and large bowel, and the genitourinary system, along with most of their accompanying blood vessels – can be visualised with ultrasound. This allows the trained critical care practitioner to use focused abdominal sonography to

- Identify causes of acute shock: Examine the aorta for signs of a ruptured aneurysm, identify free intra-abdominal fluid on a Focused Abdominal Sonography in Trauma (FAST) scan.
- Identify causes of an acute abdomen: cholecystitis, intra-abdominal abscesses, small bowel obstruction, appendicitis, pancreatitis and gastric perforation can be identified.
- Assess causes of low urine output, in particular ruling in (or out) an obstructed urinary tract (Figures 23.7 and 23.8).

VASCULAR ULTRASOUND

All vascular devices – central venous catheters, arterial lines, peripheral venous catheters, peripherally inserted central catheters (PICCs) and even ECMO catheters and intra-aortic balloon pumps – can be inserted with ultrasound guidance.

Ultrasound allows initial assessment and selection of a suitable vessel, real-time observation of the procedure, optimisation of line position, and assessment for post-procedure complications. The use of ultrasound to guide a central venous catheter is now established practice (NICE guidelines), although it does not negate the need for sound knowledge of the underlying anatomy (Figure 23.9).

Venous thromboembolic disease is an area of caution for the critical care practitioner. Despite regular prophylaxis, 8% of patients still experience this

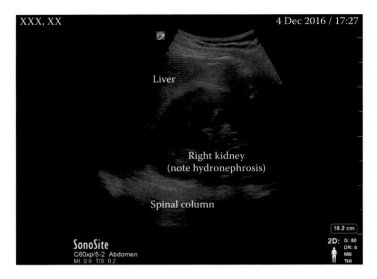

Figure 23.7 Right FAST view. Right hydronephrosis is noted.

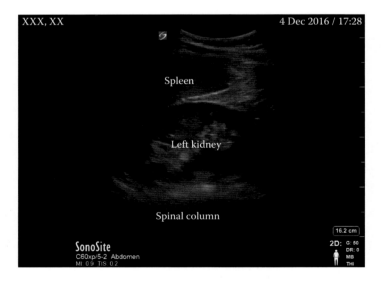

Figure 23.8 Left FAST view.

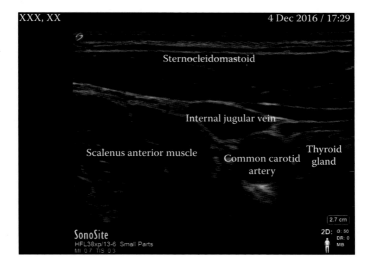

Figure 23.9 View of left internal jugular vein.

complication. Ultrasound once again proves useful in diagnosing deep vein thrombosis. A graded compression technique, when used properly, will identify the vast majority of both upper and lower limb DVTs.

HOW WOULD ULTRASOUND HELP OUR PATIENT?

The patient above is shocked, hypoxic and oliguric. Considering the history, the differential diagnosis would include multi-organ failure due to sepsis from a community-acquired pneumonia. As described above, ultrasound examination can be exceedingly useful.

Echocardiography would allow for rapid assessment of fluid status and ventricular function. This would allow us to diagnose which category of shock he falls into. Although patients with sepsis often present in hypovolaemic shock, echocardiography would rule out (or in) septic cardiomyopathy as a cause for his poor perfusion. Following on from this, it would allow the clinician to assess his response to fluid challenges.

A lung ultrasound is much more sensitive at diagnosing consolidation compared to plain radiographs. An examination using ultrasound would also allow for the detection and sampling of pleural effusion in order to aid the diagnosis. Other causes of hypoxia, such as pulmonary embolus, could be actively sought and assessed for.

This patient is almost certainly going to have a degree of acute kidney injury. Part of workup in such a situation is to rule out hydronephrosis as a cause for his oliguria (as recommended by KDIGO guidelines).

If he fails to improve with fluid therapy, ultrasound would prove useful in inserting central venous and arterial lines for continual monitoring. Serial heart and lung ultrasounds would prove helpful in assessing his response to inotropes, and assessing for signs of fluid overload. Hopefully this would prevent him from having a cardiac arrest. Yet, if he did, ultrasound would be very useful in identifying the cause (hypovolaemia, pulmonary embolus, pneumothorax, tamponade, or cardiogenic shock) and directing treatment. If he required intubation on ICU, ultrasound could help optimise his ventilation and identify when he would be ready to wean from ventilatory support.

KEY LEARNING POINTS

- Ultrasound is an imaging modality involving the use of high-frequency sound waves. Transmitting and receiving the reflections of the waves off tissue allows an image to be displayed and interpreted in real time.
- Cardiac, lung, abdominal and vascular ultrasound are the common modalities used in critical care.
- Ultrasound can be used in diagnosis – especially in shock states, to aid procedures such as lines insertion, and in assessing the clinical response to therapies.

FURTHER READING

Intensive Care Society "Resources | FICE & CUSIC | CUSIC." www.ics.ac.uk /ICS/cusic.aspx.

Lichtenstein, Daniel A. Whole Body Ultrasonography in the Critically Ill. London: Springer Publishing, 2010.

National Institute for Health and Care Excellence. "Guidelines on the Use of Ultrasound Locating Devices for Placing Central Venous Catheters." Technology appraisal guidance TA49, National Institute for Health and Care Excellence, Manchester, UK, October 2002 (updated September 2016). www.nice.org.uk/guidance/ta49.

Via, Gabriele, Arif Hussain, Mike Wells, Robert Reardon, Mahmoud ElBarbary, Vicki E. Noble, James W. Tsung, Aleksandar N. Neskovic, Susanna Price, Achikam Oren-Grinberg, Andrew Liteplo, Ricardo Cordioli, Nitha Naqvi, Philippe Rola, Jan Poelaert, Tatjana Golob Guliĉ, Erik Sloth, Arthur Labovitz, Bruce Kimura, Raoul Breitkreutz, Navroz Masani, Justin Bowra, Daniel Talmor, Fabio Guarracino, Adrian Goudie, Wang Xiaoting, Rajesh Chawla, Maurizio Galderisi, Micheal Blaivas, Tomislav Petrovic, Enrico Storti, Luca Neri, and Lawrence Melniker, for the International Conference on Focused Cardiac UltraSound (IC-FoCUS). "International Evidence-Based Recommendations for Focused Cardiac Ultrasound." *Journal of the American Society of Echocardiography* 27, no. 7 (July 2014): 683e1–683e33.

24

Renal replacement therapy in intensive care

AOIFE ABBEY AND NITIN ARORA

Mr Smith was admitted to intensive care with sepsis and hypotension. He has only passed 20 mL of urine over the past three hours and the potassium on his last blood gas was 6.8 mmol/L. He had some insulin and dextrose earlier on this evening but it doesn't seem to help for very long. What should we do next?

While there are lots of different conditions where renal replacement therapy (RRT) might be required in intensive care, the basic indications for starting this treatment are relatively defined and straightforward:

1. Acute kidney injury
    a. Hyperkalaemia (usually more than 6.5 mmoL/L)
    b. Uraemia
    c. Metabolic acidosis
    d. Evidence of fluid overload
2. Overdose of drugs or substances amenable to dialysis
    a. Drugs that can be removed by RRT are usually soluble in water and not highly protein-bound.
    b. Examples include lithium, salicylates, ethylene glycol (used in antifreeze) and methanol.

> *If you have a head for mnemonics, you might remember HUME as associated with Dr David M. Hume, an American surgeon who is co-credited with the first successful human renal transplantation in 1945.*

TYPES OF RENAL REPLACEMENT THERAPY

In intensive care, we use RRT that works by passing blood through an extracorporeal circuit where filtration, dialysis or a combination of both occurs.

It is worth taking time to understand the difference between haemo*dialysis* and haemo*filtration*.

DIALYSIS

- Occurs mainly by *diffusion* (recall Fick's law).
- Blood is pumped from the patient into the extracorporeal circuit, where it runs in the opposite direction to a dialysate fluid, separated by a semi-permeable membrane. This is called a 'countercurrent mechanism'.
- Solutes move in and out of the blood and dialysate according to their concentration gradients.

- The countercurrent mechanism ensures that a concentration gradient is maintained throughout the circuit.
- The circuit uses a pump to move both blood and dialysate through it. To remove fluid volume from a patient, pressure is used to force water across the membrane into the dialysate.

FILTRATION

- Occurs mainly by *convection* (solvent drag).
- Blood is pumped from the patient into the extracorporeal circuit, where it runs along a semipermeable membrane.
- The hydrostatic pressure on the blood side of the circuit creates a trans-membrane pressure, which forces fluid and molecules that are small enough across the membrane.
- This is called ultrafiltration and is similar to the mechanism of glomerular filtration, which occurs between the glomerulus and Bowman's capsule.
- Unlike in a real kidney, after filtration all of the ultrafiltrate is discarded and both volume and electrolytes are replaced with a sort of idealized plasma called 'filtration fluid'.

INTERMITTENT RRT

You might be familiar with intermittent haemodialysis. This is the type of treatment patients with end-stage renal failure get for 3–5 hours three times a week.

In order for sufficient dialysis and fluid removal to occur in this short time, it is necessary to use relatively high pressure though the circuit. Typical blood flow required is 200–400 mL/min. Dialysate is pumped through the circuit at 500–800 mL/min.

While this means that intermittent RRT is highly efficient, it usually felt unsuited to haemodynamically unstable patients and is not widely used within the intensive care setting.

In-patients with acute kidney injury who are otherwise stable can also have intermittent haemodialysis outside of an ICU/HDU setting under the supervision of the renal team.

CONTINUOUS RRT (CRRT)

Continuous RRT uses lower pressures and works slowly over a longer time. It is less efficient, but can be used on sick, unstable patients and is the common choice of RRT on intensive care.

There are different types of continuous RRT. They sound complicated and can seem overwhelming, but they are all essentially just dialysis, filtration or a combination of both.

In the past, arterio-venous circuits, which used the patient's own blood pressure to drive blood through the system, were used. This method has now been abandoned in favour of veno-venous circuits. In contrast to intermittent therapy, the flow of blood is slower (typically 50–200 mL/min).

- **CVVHD = Continuous veno-venous haemodialysis**
  - This is really slow dialysis (as described above).
  - Solute removal is controlled by the type of dialysate fluid used.
  - At low flow rates, there is no fluid removed (not enough pressure).
- **CVVHF = Continuous veno-venous haemofiltration**
  - This is slow filtration (as described above).
  - Both solute and fluid is removed.
  - The filtered fluid (ultrafiltrate) is removed and then replacement fluid added according to what is required.
- **CVVHDF = Continuous veno-venous haemodiafiltration**
  - This is a combination of both CVVHF and CVVHD.
- **SCUF = Slow continuous ultrafiltration**
  - This is really slow, low pressure CVVHF and is used when the only requirement is fluid removal.

SUSTAINED LOW EFFICIENCY DIALYSIS (SLED) (OR SLEDD: SLOW LOW EFFICIENCY DAILY DIALYSIS)

- SLED employs a mechanism that is a hybrid between intermittent and continuous RRT and occurs over 6–12 hours.
- The proposed benefit of SLED is that it is as effective at solute removal as continuous RRT, but it is a more time and cost efficient treatment for

patients that would not tolerate the haemodynamic demands of intermittent haemodialysis.

- Blood flow will typically be 200–300 mL/min.

SO HOW DO WE PICK?

- An intensive care unit may choose to chiefly use CCVHF, CVVHD, CVVHDF or SLED but their choice is likely to reflect established preferences and local factors including equipment availability, new funding and nurse training.
- There is no firm evidence that any particular method of continuous RRT based on filtration or dialysis is superior in terms of patient survival or recovery of renal function.
- Although not common, there are some intensive care units in the UK who use intermittent haemodialysis to good effect.

VASCULAR ACCESS

In intensive care, we now exclusively use veno-venous RRT. This is carried out using a type of venous central line called a 'vascath'.

Flow is better through large, central veins and so the aim is to have the catheter tip inside the vena cava. Potential sites of access are therefore the subclavian or internal jugular veins, which allow access to the superior vena cava, or the femoral vein, which allows access into the inferior vena cava.

A vascath is made up of two lumens: a proximal (red) lumen, which takes blood out of the patient into the machine; and a distal (blue) lumen, which is the site of return.

ANTICOAGULATION

Blood flowing through the circuit is liable to clot. You might hear a nurse tell you that their filter has 'come down' or 'clotted off'. If a circuit clots off completely, the blood within the circuit is lost to the patient. This can be up to 250 mL of blood! Clotted circuits are also a problem because putting up a new circuit interrupts treatment, has a financial cost and takes up nursing time.

To decrease the probability of this occurrence, we anticoagulate the circuit. The most common choice in UK intensive care units is unfractionated heparin. Low molecular weight heparin, citrate and prostaglandins can also be used.

Although the aim is to anticoagulate the circuit, rather than the patient, there are patient factors that would preclude the use of anticoagulation. These include a high INR, high APTT, low platelet count or other high bleeding risk.

CONCEPTS IN PRESCRIBING CRRT

The majority of UK intensive care units use CVVHF as the first choice of continuous RRT in their patients. A typical prescription for CVVHF should consider:

ANTICOAGULATION

- Circuit primed usually with 5000 units of heparin in 1000 mL 0.9% sodium chloride (not delivered to patient).
- The first-choice anticoagulant is generally unfractionated heparin at a rate of 5–10 units/kg/hr according to bleeding risk.
- Some units now use RRT circuits that can use citrate as an anticoagulant.

EXCHANGE RATE

- For CVVHF, this is simply the amount of ultrafiltration per kilogramme of bodyweight per hour. It is sometimes referred to as the rate of effluent production.
- Normal range is 25–35 mL/kg/hr.

FLUID REPLACEMENT AND BALANCE

- If a 70-kg patient is having CVVHF at an exchange rate of 30 mL/kg/hr, the ultrafiltrate made in one hour is 2100 mL. This is then replaced by a type of idealized plasma called 'filtration fluid'.

- If part of the volume of ultrafiltrate made is not replaced, then this amounts to fluid removal.
- The amount of fluid removed is determined by overall fluid balance and clinical examination.
- A patient's ability to tolerate fluid removal is dependent on their haemodynamic stability but typical rates are 50–400 mL/hr.

REPLACEMENT FLUID CHOICE

- Replacement fluid is buffered with either lactate or bicarbonate.
- Although a healthy person will readily metabolise lactate into bicarbonate, this ability may be impaired in the critically unwell patient and the majority of fluid used is now lactate free.
- The amount of potassium in the replacement fluid should also be considered.

PRE- AND POST-DILUTION

- The fluid that ultimately replaces the ultrafiltrate can be added into the circuit either before or after the filter.
- Pre-filter dilution has the benefit of diluting the blood before filtration, which can increase the life of the filter by preventing clotting.
- Pre-filter dilution can also be used to augment blood flow rate, which will ultimately determine filtration rate.
- The trade off to pre-filter dilution is that less concentrated blood dilutes solutes and can adversely affect clearance. You also need larger amounts of fluid for pre-filter dilution.
- Standard practice is to use a combination of both, usually starting with a 30% pre- and 70% post-dilution fraction.

WHAT ARE YOU GOING TO DO FOR MR SMITH?

You review Mr Smith and agree he is oliguric. You examine his fluid status and see this is despite adequate fluid resuscitation and blood pressure support with noradrenaline, his overall fluid balance is 3000 mL positive.

You look at his blood gas and see that he also has a metabolic acidosis with a high potassium level. These are criteria for renal replacement therapy.

You feel that because he is a haemodynamically unstable and acutely unwell patient, continuous RRT is the most appropriate option and that he will require venous access via a vascath to start CRRT. You advise the nurse to aim for an overall negative fluid balance of 1500 mL over the next 24 hours.

FURTHER READING

Bellomo, Rinaldo, and Claudio Ronco. "Continuous Renal Replacement Therapy: Hemofiltration, Hemodiafiltration or Hemodialysis." In *Critical Care Nephrology*, 2nd edition, edited by Claudio Ronco, Rinaldo Bellomo, and John A. Kellum. 1354–1358. Philadelphia: Saunders Elsevier, 2009.

Intensive Care Society. "Standards and Recommendations for the Provision of Renal Replacement Therapy on Intensive Care Units in the UK." 2009. www.ics.ac.uk/ICS/guidelines-and-standards.aspx (accessed 12 April 2016).

RENAL Replacement Therapy Study Investigators. "Intensity of Continuous Renal-Replacement Therapy in Critically Ill Patients." *New England Journal of Medicine* 361, no. 17 (October 2009): 1627–1638.

Ronco, Claudio, Zaccaria Ricci, Daniel De Backer, John A. Kellum, Fabio S. Taccone, Michael Joannidis, Peter Pickkers, Vincenzo Cantaluppi, Franco Turani, Patrick Saudan, Rinaldo Bellomo, Olivier Joannes-Boyau, Massimo Antonelli, Didier Payen, John R. Prowle, and Jean-Louis Vincent. "Renal Replacement Therapy in Acute Kidney Injury: Controversy and Consensus." *Critical Care* 19, no. 1 (2015): 146.

Vijayan, Anitha. "Vascular Access for Continuous Renal Replacement Therapy." *Seminars in Dialysis* 22, no. 2 (2009): 133–136.

25

Interpreting arterial blood gases (ABGs)

NAFEESA AKHTAR AND JULIAN HULL

'*Mrs Norma Lenilas is looking unwell. She came in with COPD. She hasn't eaten all weekend so we have given plenty of IV fluids. Her breathing has deteriorated, and she looks tired…*

I have done a blood gas test; here are the results.

pH	*7.19*
PaCO₂	*5.22*
pO₂	*8.07*
HCO₃⁻	*14.9*
Lac	*1.8*
BE	*−13.1*
Cl⁻	*122.2*
K⁺	*4.6*
Na⁺	*144.7*

What should we do?'

This is a familiar phone call, which you could receive at any time when covering Critical Care.

Key things to consider when given a similar history and blood results are

- What type of abnormality is present – respiratory and/or metabolic?
- What does it mean?
- What should your immediate management involve?

WHAT IS AN ABG?

An ABG (arterial blood gas) analyser primarily measures the hydrogen ion concentration (pH) and blood gas tension or partial pressure of oxygen (PaO_2) and carbon dioxide ($PaCO_2$) dissolved in the blood and then calculates other components of acid base status.

Other blood components are frequently also measured, though are not strictly part of blood gas analysis (see below).

NORMAL VALUES FOR ARTERIAL BLOOD GAS (ABG)

Below are normal ranges. These values are usually documented on the printout along with the patient's ABG results.

- pH: 7.35–7.45
- pO_2: 10–14 kPa
- $PaCO_2$: 4.5–6 kPa

- Base excess (BE): -2 ± 2 mmol L^{-1}
- HCO_3^-: 22–26 mmol L^{-1}

Note: 1 kPa = approximately 7.5 mmHg.

DEFINITIONS

pH – is the negative logarithm (to base 10) of hydrogen ion (H^+) concentration. Outside the normal values, a low pH indicates a high H^+ concentration, and an acidosis. Conversely, a high pH indicates a low H^+ concentration, and therefore an alkalotic state.

pH is tightly controlled between 7.35–7.45, by the buffering capacity of the body.

The major buffers include:

- Intracellular: Proteins, particularly haemoglobin, phosphate
- Extracellular: Bicarbonate, proteins and phosphate
- Urine: Ammonia and phosphate
- Bone: In chronic acidotic states

Acid load is removed by

- The lungs (exhaled CO_2) – if this is ineffective, it will produce a respiratory acidosis.
- The kidneys (excreted H^+ ions) – if this is overwhelmed, a metabolic acidosis will result.

It is important to note that if a state of acidosis or alkalosis is compensated for, the pH may be near normal.

Partial pressure – in a mixture of gases, it is the pressure a gas would exert if it alone occupied the same volume. In a solution (e.g. blood), this pressure (or tension) is equal to the pressure the gas would exert in a gas phase in equilibrium with the liquid. This is often termed the partial pressure of the gas in blood.

The letter 'a' is added to denote arterial blood, as opposed to 'v' indicating venous blood.

- pO_2 – the partial pressure of oxygen in arterial blood, PaO_2
- pCO_2 – the partial pressure of carbon dioxide in arterial blood, $PaCO_2$

Actual bicarbonate is the concentration of bicarbonate (HCO_3^-) in the blood. The bicarbonate concentration is derived from the Henderson–Hasselbalch equation.

$$pH = pK + \log \frac{[\text{bicarbonate}]}{[\text{carbon dioxide}]}$$

Standard bicarbonate is the HCO_3^- concentration when respiratory changes are eliminated by deriving the value under standard conditions of $PaCO_2$ (5.3 kPa), temperature (37°C), and fully oxygenated blood.

Base excess is the amount of alkali that would be required (added or removed) to return the pH of *in vitro blood* to 7.4, again under standard conditions of $PaCO_2$, temperature and fully oxygenated blood. Like standard bicarbonate, it reflects metabolic, as opposed to respiratory, acid/base changes.

Standard base excess is the amount of alkali that would be required to return the pH of extracellular fluid to 7.4, under standard conditions. This is thought to better reflect in-vivo changes.

Normal values are between −2 and +2 mEq L^{-1}.

- More negative than −2 (deficit) indicates a metabolic acidosis.
- More positive than +2 (excess) indicates a metabolic acidosis.

OTHER COMPONENTS

Blood gas analysis can now give us much more information, including:

Lactate – a by-product of anaerobic respiration, a raised level can be due to poor tissue perfusion.

Glucose – very helpful in an emergency, or when monitoring a critically unwell patient.

Electrolytes – usually potassium, sodium, calcium and chloride. Again helpful in an emergency, especially with dysrhythmias and in fluid management.

Anion Gap – the calculated difference between the measured anions and cations, and can be helpful when considering the many causes of metabolic acidosis.

$$\text{Anion Gap} = \left[Na^+\right] + \left[K^+\right] - \left[Cl^-\right] - \left[HCO_3^-\right]$$

Approximate reference range 4–16 mmol L^{-1}. High values indicate the possibility of additional unmeasured acids.

Haemoglobin (Hb) – not always accurate, but helpful to follow trends.

Carbon Monoxide (CO) – If your analyser has a co-oximeter, the carboxy-haemoglobin (HbCO) level is shown as a percentage. Raised levels may be present in smokers, and in cases of CO poisoning.

Methaemoglobin (MetHb) – an oxidised form of Hb. Normal levels are less than 2%. Levels may be elevated due to congenital enzyme deficiencies, or due to the use of drugs such as antibiotics (trimethoprim, sulphonamides) and local anaesthetics (prilocaine).

ALTERNATIVE APPROACHES TO BLOOD GAS ANALYSIS

In the 1980s, Canadian physiologist Peter Stewart proposed an alternative approach to acid–base physiology using the physicochemical laws of mass action, conservation of mass and electrical neutrality. The traditional Henderson–Hasselbalch equation-based approach has limitations beyond respiratory derived acid–base disturbances. Stewart's concept of strong ions (Na^+, K^+, Mg^{2+}, Ca^{2+}, SO_4^{2-}, Cl^-), which are in plasma concentrations in the order of a million times more than H^+ (normal, 40 nanomoles L^{-1}), allows for the calculation of the Strong Ion Difference (SID). Together with other independent variables, $PaCO_2$ and total weak acid, the SID can be used to calculate the pH and give information about non-respiratory acid–base disturbances. The Stewart approach is not used routinely in most ICUs.

HOW TO INTERPRET AN ABG

WHAT IS THE PO_2?

- Is oxygenation adequate? Take into consideration how much oxygen the patient was breathing (FiO_2) when the ABG was taken.
- One way of relating the resulting PaO_2 from varying amounts of inspired oxygen is to determine the PaO_2/FiO_2 ratio, (often called the 'P to F ratio'). This can help to determine whether an improvement in PaO_2 is

due to improving lung function or a change in ventilator settings, or simply due to an increased FiO_2. For example, if somebody has a pO_2 of 13 kPa on 21% oxygen, the ratio would be

- $13/0.21 = 61.9$

WHAT IS THE pH?

- Is the pH within the normal range?
- If not, is there an acidosis or alkalosis present?
- Could there be a mixed picture of acidosis *and* alkalosis or is there some compensation?

IS THE pH CHANGE DUE TO A PRIMARY RESPIRATORY OR METABOLIC DISTURBANCE? CHECK THE $PaCO_2$ AND HCO_3^-

Primary respiratory and metabolic changes have the following characteristics:

- Respiratory acidosis – high $PaCO_2$ and normal to high HCO_3^- (metabolic compensation)
- Respiratory alkalosis – low $PaCO_2$ and normal to low HCO_3^- (metabolic compensation)
- Metabolic acidosis – low HCO_3^- and normal to low $PaCO_2$ (respiratory compensation)
- Metabolic alkalosis – high HCO_3^- and normal to high $PaCO_2$ (respiratory compensation)
- Note that secondary respiratory and metabolic compensatory changes normally do not fully compensate for the primary disturbance

If the $PaCO_2$ and HCO_3^- trend in opposite directions, it may suggest a mixed disorder.

WHAT IS THE BASE EXCESS AND ANION GAP?

A negative (< −2) base excess indicates metabolic acidosis. The anion gap can give further information about the underlying cause.

- Normal anion gap – Causes include renal tubular acidosis, renal compensation for respiratory alkalosis, electrolyte losses due to diarrhoea or hyperchloraemic acidosis due to saline infusion.
- High anion gap – Causes include ketoacidosis, lactic acidosis, renal failure or toxins.
  A positive (> +2) base excess indicates a metabolic alkalosis.
- Causes include renal reabsorption of bicarbonate, or compensation for a respiratory acidosis.

Note hypoalbuminaemia can cause a low anion gap by reducing the body's overall anion proportion.

IS THERE EVIDENCE OF COMPENSATION?

- The classic example of this is a patient with COPD with a raised baseline $PaCO_2$, for which the body has compensated by raising the HCO_3^- to counter the respiratory acidosis and normalise the pH.
- Or in case of a metabolic acidosis in which a patient hyperventilates in order to 'blow off' carbon dioxide and so lower the $PaCO_2$.

But remember… look at your patient! Ask yourself does your interpretation of the ABG fit with the clinical picture? Review the history and examination findings.

WHAT SHOULD WE DO?

Picking up from the very last point, we would need to assess our patient; receive a handover, take a history and examine Mrs Lenilas.

Norma is a 60-year-old lady, who had been admitted four days ago with an infective exacerbation of COPD, and has become more breathless over the last 48 hours. Worried about sepsis, a keen junior had prescribed for her 7 litres of normal saline.

Now considering key information from the ABG:

- pO_2 8.07 – Is this oxygenation adequate? The immediate problem is we do not know how much oxygen Norma was on when this was taken. This is a low value, but if it was taken on 15 L O_2, we would be very worried!
- pH 7.19 – indicating acidosis.

- $PaCO_2$ 5.22 and HCO_3^- 14.9 – normal $PaCO_2$ and low HCO_3^-, indicating a metabolic acidosis.
- BE –13.1 – this is very low.
  - Considering the anion gap:
  - $(Na^+ 144.7 + K^+ 4.6)–(HCO_3^- 14.9 + Cl^- 122.2) = 12.2$, therefore normal.
- There does not appear to be any compensation.
- Of the other components in the analysis, the Cl^- is raised.

Overall, this would suggest an uncompensated iatrogenic hyperchloraemic metabolic acidosis, caused by excessive 0.9% NaCl infusion.

IMMEDIATE MANAGEMENT

Remember your ABC approach.

- Ensure the airway is patent, and give oxygen as required.
- If improved oxygenation is required with support, consider non-invasive ventilation.
- Ensure suitable venous access. In this case, Norma may be 'well filled' but require alternative fluids.
- Consider diuretics if excessive fluids have been given during resuscitation, bearing in mind how this may further alter the electrolyte load.
- If the acidosis is slow to correct and complicated by organ failure, renal replacement therapy may be necessary.

KEY LEARNING POINTS

- An ABG can be used to assess adequacy of ventilation and assess the acid base status for a patient.
- Due to the speed of results, this test is very helpful in an emergency. Remember if you cannot gain an arterial blood gas, a venous or capillary sample can be invaluable.
- Use a systematic approach when interpreting an ABG.
- Always assess your patient and never treat an ABG result in isolation!

FURTHER READING

Brandis, Kerry. *Acid-Base pHysiology*. Online textbook. www.anaesthesiamcq
.com/AcidBaseBook (accessed 28 January 2017).Key Learning Points

Cadogan, Mike, and Chris Nickson. "Life in the Fast Lane: Acid Base Disorders."
http://lifeinthefastlane.com/investigations/acid-base/(accessed 28 January
2017).

Grogono, Alan W. 2016. "Acid-Base Tutorial: Stewart's Strong Ion Difference."
www.acid-base.com/strongion.php (accessed 28 January 2017).

Lloyd, Peter. "Strong Ion Calculator – A Practical Bedside Application
of Modern Quantitative Acid-Base Physiology." *Critical Care and
Resuscitation* 6 (2004): 285–294. www.cicm.org.au/CICM_Media
/CICMSite/CICM-Website/Resources/Publications/CCR%20Journal
/Previous%20Editions/December%202004/12_2004_Dec_Strong-Ion
-Calculator.pdf (accessed 28 January 2017).

Oxford Medical Education. 2017. "Arterial Blood Gas (ABG) Interpretation for Medical Students, OSCES and MRCP PACES." www.oxfordmedicaleducation
.com/abgs/abg-interpretation/(accessed 28 January 2017).

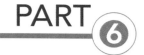

PART 6

AIRWAY AND RESPIRATORY EMERGENCIES

26

Maintaining an airway

VIJAY VENKATESH AND NITIN ARORA

The nurse asks you to urgently review a patient whose consciousness has decreased and has developed noisy breathing.

Maintaining an airway is a life-saving procedure with which all doctors should be familiar. Though airway experts are part of the crash call team, the staff in the ward are expected to manage the airway until help arrives.

CAUSES OF AIRWAY OBSTRUCTION

Obstruction of the upper airways may be partial or complete. In the unconscious patient, this is generally due to loss of pharyngeal muscle tone. It may also be caused by vomit, blood from trauma, or by a foreign body.

Laryngeal obstruction may be caused by trauma, inflammation or burns.

RECOGNISING AN OBSTRUCTED AIRWAY

- This is best managed by the look, listen and feel approach.
- **Look** for chest and abdomen movements.
- **Listen** and **feel** for air coming out of the mouth and nose, and for any added sounds.
- Added sounds may be due to partial airway obstruction, and may include stridor, gurgling or snoring.

BASIC AIRWAY OPENING MANOEUVRES

After recognising airway obstruction, the next step is to relieve it. The main manoeuvres used are as follows:

- Head tilt
- Chin lift
- Jaw thrust

HEAD TILT AND CHIN LIFT

Place one hand on the patient's forehead, and use the other hand to gently lift the chin. This is generally successful, but must not be attempted if there is cervical spine instability, in which case the jaw thrust technique should be tried.

JAW THRUST

Locate the angle of the mandible and then, with the fingers under the angle, apply upward pressure while opening the mouth with the thumbs.

Reassess the airway by looking, listening and feeling after each manoeuvre, to assess success.

If a clear airway is not achieved, look for other causes of obstruction (e.g. foreign bodies, vomit, etc.).

AIRWAY ADJUNCTS

If the above basic techniques have not been successful, oropharyngeal or nasopharyngeal airways may be tried.

The oropharyngeal (Guedel) airway is a curved plastic tube with a flange at the end. It must be sized appropriately before insertion. Its length should be the distance between the patient's incisors and the angle of the jaw. For insertion of this device, open the mouth and insert the airway 'upside down' until it reaches the soft palate. Rotate it through 180° and then advance it again until it is in the pharynx. The flattened portion should sit between the patient's teeth. After insertion, reassess the airway as described above.

The nasopharyngeal airway is a soft plastic tube with a bevel at one end and a flange at the other. It is better tolerated than the Guedel airway by patients who are not deeply unconscious. Sizes 6–7 are suitable for most adults. Lubricate the airway and then insert the airway gently into the nose with a twisting motion.

This airway must not be used in a suspected base-of-skull fracture. Extreme caution should be exercised in patients prone for bleeding owing to vascularity of nasal mucosa.

Once the airway is in place, reassess it as described earlier.

Chin lift, head tilt and jaw thrust may still be needed in conjunction with these airways.

VENTILATION

If the patient is not breathing despite an open airway, artificial ventilation must be started. Mouth-to-mouth and pocket-mask ventilation are options, but in a hospital setting you would generally have access to a self-inflating bag and mask. We recommend a two-person technique where one person holds the mask on the patient's face with jaw thrust while the assistant squeezes the bag. This enables a better seal and more effective ventilation.

Using a bag and mask requires skill and practice, but can be extremely useful for resuscitation.

ADVANCED AIRWAYS

Laryngeal mask airways (LMA) and endotracheal tubes provide a better airway with more effective ventilation, but discussion of their insertion and use is beyond the scope of this book.

APPROACHING THE ABOVE CLINICAL PROBLEM

- Recognise whether the airway is obstructed by look, listen and feel as explained above. Expert help should be sought immediately once airway obstruction is confirmed.
- Airway manoeuvres like head tilt and chin lift to open the obstructed airway; jaw thrust may be required. At this point, make sure the obstruction is not because of blood, secretions, vomitus or foreign body. Also, administer high flow oxygen to be given via a non-rebreathe mask.
- If obstruction does not improve, airway adjuncts like oropharyngeal or nasopharyngeal airway are to be inserted.
- Next step is to try and ventilate the patient with bag and mask with a two-person technique.
- This patient is likely to require advanced airway insertion but the decision and insertion of these are the responsibility of airway experts.

Every doctor should be able to perform basic airway management. This skill will be very useful when airway emergencies happen in areas where airway experts are not immediately available.

27

Rapid sequence induction

SUDHINDRA KULKARNI AND SHONDIPON K. LAHA

*'Miss Thomas is a 32-year-old female patient with a suspected head injury and a GCS of 9. Her partner says she has eaten an hour ago and she needs **airway protection** for safe conduct of a CT scan and further decision for possible transfer to a tertiary neurosurgical centre.'*

This is a common scenario one faces being on call for the intensive care unit (ICU).

Rapid sequence induction, or rapid sequence intubation (RSI) is an established method of inducing anaesthesia in patients who are at risk of aspiration of gastric contents into the lungs. The basic principle is intubation of the trachea during application of cricoid pressure following loss of consciousness. The main objective of the technique is to minimise the time interval between loss of protective airway reflexes and tracheal intubation with a cuffed endotracheal tube. Because the airway is unprotected during this time, it is the most critical period during which aspiration of gastric contents is likely to occur.

INDICATIONS

During emergency intubation, aspiration of stomach contents is a potential risk in all patients with an incompetent larynx. Pre-intubation fasting and pro-kinetic agents reduce this risk but are not always appropriate or available before emergency intubation and ventilation.

The Royal College of Anaesthetists National Audit Project (NAP4) recommended an RSI with cricoid pressure of the technique of choice to induce anaesthesia in those patients at risk of regurgitation and subsequent aspiration.

RISK OF PROCEDURE

RSI as a practice is not without risk, particularly in the critically ill patients. Risks include hypoxia, failed intubation, oesophageal trauma, cardiovascular compromise and awareness.

Many factors influence the degree of risk (Figure 27.1).

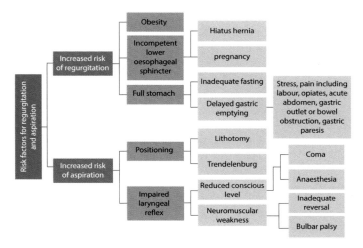

Figure 27.1 Risk factors for regurgitation and aspiration.

HOW TO DO AN RSI

Essential features in the performance of an RSI are remembered as the 9Ps:

- Planning
- Preparation (drugs, equipment, people, place)
- Protect the cervical spine
- Positioning (some do this after paralysis and induction)
- Pre-oxygenation
- Pressure – Cricoid
- Paralysis and Induction
- Placement confirmation with capnography
- Post-intubation management

MINIMIZING ASPIRATION RISK

CRICOID PRESSURE

Cricoid pressure describes the backward displacement of the complete cartilaginous cricoid ring against the cervical vertebrae to occlude the hypopharynx. The technique usually involves the application of a 10-N force before induction, increasing this force to 30 N on loss of consciousness. It should be removed immediately if active vomiting occurs as there is a risk of oesophageal rupture.

The NAP4 guidelines support use of cricoid pressure as part of an RSI and is considered a standard of care in the UK. This should be supported by adequate training and practice in its use. There should be a low threshold for reducing or removing cricoid pressure if intubation or mask ventilation proves difficult and to facilitate LMA insertion or cricothyroidotomy rescue techniques.

TRACHEAL INTUBATION

A cuffed tracheal tube represents the gold standard in airway protection and should be used in Rapid Sequence Intubation. After a failed RSI, where mask ventilation is difficult or impossible, the use of a supraglottic airway device (SAD) is recommended. The use of a second-generation SAD in this situation, with its superior seal pressure to facilitate assisted ventilation and the presence of a channel to direct gastric contents away from the larynx, makes particular sense. Similarly, in a 'can't intubate, can't ventilate' scenario requiring cricothyroidotomy, there is a strong argument for performing a surgical airway and inserting a cuffed tracheal tube that will provide both oxygenation and airway protection.

OPTIMIZING OXYGENATION PRIOR TO INTUBATION

ADEQUATE PREOXYGENATION

Preoxygenation is an attempt to maximize oxygen stores in the body before a period of pharmacologically induced apnoea. The majority of these stores are contained within the lungs as part of the functional residual capacity (FRC). Critically ill patients with high metabolic rates, low cardiac outputs, and respiratory pathology and patients with a reduced FRC, such as the obese and the parturient, have a lower oxygen storage capacity and will desaturate more rapidly.

INCREASE F_IO_2

Evidence shows that 3–5 minutes of tidal ventilation with 100% oxygen, ensuring a tight mask fit and high gas flows, will maximize denitrogenation. This practice is particularly very important in critically ill patients who can very rapidly desaturate due to minimal reserves.

POSITIVE PRESSURE

Positive end-expiratory pressure (PEEP) and continuous positive airway pressure (CPAP) have been shown to reduce absorption atelectasis, improve PaO_2, and increase time to desaturation in all patient groups. If a patient is already receiving non-invasive ventilation (NIV) or has a degree of respiratory compromise, the evidence suggests that continuing or commencing NIV for a short period while setting up for intubation is better protection against desaturation than standard preoxygenation.

NIV in obese surgical patients specifically has been shown to improve preoxygenation. Concerns about increasing aspiration by gastric distension can be balanced by adopting upright positioning to reduce the risk of passive regurgitation and by limiting airway pressures. Gastric distension and regurgitation risk are low if pressures are kept below 25 cmH_2O.

APNOEIC OXYGENATION

As a result of differences in solubility of O_2 and CO_2, once the patient is apnoeic, more O_2 leaves the alveoli and enters the bloodstream than CO_2 or N_2 enter it, creating a slightly negative pressure (increasing atelectasis). This negative pressure can be used to an advantage by maintaining a patent airway and continuing administration of oxygen that then reaches the alveoli by bulk flow. The application of nasal prongs or humidified high flow nasal oxygen in addition to face mask oxygen allows this process to continue during laryngoscopy and has been shown to increase time to desaturation after apnoea in both normal and obese surgical populations.

POSITIONING FOR PREOXYGENATION

FRC is lower in the supine position. Evidence in normal, obese, and pregnant populations suggests that adopting a head-up position (20°–35°) increases FRC and thereby improves preoxygenation. This has been shown to be clinically significant by increasing the time from apnoea to desaturation. In patients with suspected cervical spine injury/unstable neck, it is necessary to provide the manual axial inline stabilization (MAIS) during RSI.

SUCTION EQUIPMENT AND TILTING TROLLEY

There should be a working suction apparatus with a large yankauer suction tip attached for rapid suctioning in case of vomiting and a need to clear the contents from the oropharynx and hypopharynx. A tilting trolley to facilitate a head-down position would be ideal although this may not be always available.

DRUGS IN RSI

INDUCTION AGENT

Even to date, the ideal intravenous induction agent does not exist, with individual drugs harbouring benefits and disadvantages (Table 27.1). The choice of IV induction agent should be guided by informed clinical reasoning and not by dogma. Predetermined dosing may be appropriate in those at high risk of aspiration in order to minimise the time spent with reduced protective laryngeal reflexes. This does, however, increase the risk of both under-dosing with potential awareness and also overdosing with the risk of cardiovascular collapse.

Table 27.1 The advantages and disadvantages of standard induction agents

Induction agent	Advantages	Disadvantages	Suggested use
Sodium thiopental 3–7 mg/kg (traditionally used)	Clear endpoint Rapid one arm brain circulation time	Postoperative nausea and vomiting Potential harm from extravasation Antanalgesic	Traditional choice for RSI in obstetric practice
Propofol 2–4 mg/kg (use increasing)	Greater suppression of laryngeal reflexes Familiarity	CVS depression	As an alternative to Thiopentone
Etomidate 0.3 mg/kg (use decreasing)	CVS stability	Adrenal suppression	CVS instability Caution or avoid in sepsis and, if used early, hydrocortisone recommended

(Continued)

Table 27.1 (*Continued*) The advantages and disadvantages of standard induction agents

Induction agent	Advantages	Disadvantages	Suggested use
Ketamine 1–2 mg/kg (use increasing)	Bronchodilation CVS stimulant; maintains cerebral perfusion pressure in hypotensive situations		Asthma Shocked states Being increasingly used in trauma patients
Midazolam	Not routinely used as an induction agent in the UK	Longer to take effect and long duration of action	Probably no role as a single agent
Opiate	Not routinely used as an induction agent in the UK	Unreliable amnesic. Not recommended as a general anaesthetic	Probably no role as a single agent

NEUROMUSCULAR BLOCKING AGENT

Succinylcholine is the depolarizing neuromuscular blocking agent that has traditionally been used in RSI because of its fast onset and offset, with the presumption being that, in the event of failure to intubate, ventilate or both, recovery of spontaneous ventilation would reliably rescue the situation. However, due to its relatively rapid onset and immediate reversibility, the non-depolarizing neuromuscular blocking agent rocuronium is increasingly used as an alternative.

The key issues regarding neuromuscular block (NMB) and RSI are as follows:

1. Time to complete paralysis and the quality of those intubation conditions
2. Potential reversal (spontaneous or otherwise) of this effect

3. Duration of action
4. Side effects and contraindication profile

The recommended dose of Succinylcholine is 1–2 mg/kg to provide intubation conditions. Succinylcholine as a drug has many side effects with hyperkalaemia due to potassium efflux being the most dangerous; this is increased significantly in conditions that result in up-regulation of nicotinic receptors, such as burns, crush injuries and chronic neurological conditions, including spinal cord injury, stroke and critical illness polyneuropathy. It causes malignant hyperthermia in susceptible individuals.

The recommended rocuronium dose for RSI is 1 mg/kg to provide optimal intubation conditions. Rocuronium is a relatively cleaner drug, the only absolute contraindication being allergy.

Rocuronium followed by sugammadex results in a return to spontaneous ventilation in case of failed intubation and the decision to wake up the patient. However, in RSIs in critically ill patients, 'wake up' is not a feasible option and the reversibility of the induction technique cannot be possible, for example, the patient with the ruptured abdominal aortic aneurysm or the critically ill patient with respiratory failure. In these scenarios, use of a drug that provides the best airway management conditions for more than a few minutes would seem the most effective strategy and this is also the recommendations in the new DAS guidelines.

OPIOIDS

Traditionally, opioids were not used as part of an RSI. However, the majority of intensivists use it as a part of their RSI regimen. Opioids reduce intraocular, intracranial, and cardiovascular adverse effects associated with laryngoscopy and should be considered in situations where these effects could be potentially harmful. They also reduce the dose of hypnotic agent required.

VENTILATION

Ventilation after apnoea and before intubation is traditionally avoided in RSI owing to the assumption that such practice increases gastric distension and the risk of regurgitation. In patients who have increased metabolic demands, reduced FRC, pre-existing hypoxia, respiratory pathology, or are not readily intubatable may desaturate before intubation despite adequate preoxygenation. These patients are likely to benefit from gentle ventilation with cricoid pressure applied before laryngoscopy. This has been referred to as controlled RSI.

PLANNED PREPARATION WITH CHECKLIST FOR RSI

NAP4 recommended that an intubation checklist should be developed and used for the tracheal intubations of all critically ill patients. A checklist will identify issues regarding preparation of the patient, equipment, drugs, personnel and help clarify the back-up plan. This also advocates good team working and helps the process to be smooth rather than a stressful experience. It is particularly useful for the nursing staff on ICU who may not be exposed to airway management on a regular basis unlike in a theatre environment.

We use a locally developed protocol, B@EASE (Figure 27.2).

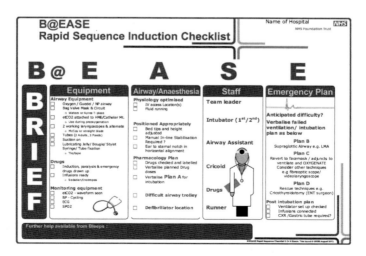

Figure 27.2 B@EASE: a rapid sequence induction checklist.

MANAGEMENT OF FAILURE – DAS GUIDELINES

The Difficult Airway Society (DAS) guidelines for the management of failed intubation and ventilation should be followed in these situations.

There should be a third person (anaesthetist, assistant or suitable alternative) present and able to summon help or retrieve the equipment required should unexpected difficulties arise. The default position in most RSIs where intubation is unsuccessful will be wake up. This may not be appropriate or possible in critically ill patients and this should be factored into the planned strategy (Figure 27.3).

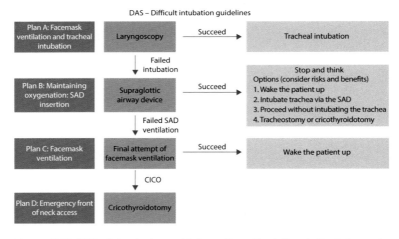

Figure 27.3 Difficult intubation guidelines. (From Frerk C et al., *Br. J. Anaesth.*, 115, 1–22, 2015. Difficult Airway Society.)

KEY LEARNING POINTS

A modified RSI as practiced in modern critical care medicine could be considered to be

- A reduction in regurgitation and aspiration risk – physical and pharmacological measures
- Assisted ventilation before intubation to maximise oxygen stores

- Application of cricoid pressure is advisable—unless it obscures the view at laryngoscopy or interferes with manual ventilation or SAD placement
- (IV) Induction of anaesthesia appropriate to clinical condition with suitable induction and NMB agents
- Planned preparation with a checklist and management of failure with DAS guidelines

FURTHER READING

B@EASE RSI Checklist. "Introducing the B@EASE Rapid Sequence Checklist." 29 September 2013. https://nwrapidsequenceinductionchecklist.wordpress .com/.

Cook, Timothy M., Nicholas Woodall, and Chris Frerk. *Major Complications of Airway Management in the United Kingdom: Report and Findings.* Fourth National Audit Project of the Royal College of Anaesthetists and Difficult Airway Society. London: Royal College of Anaesthetists, March 2011.

El-Orbany, Mohammad, and Lois A. Connolly. "Rapid Sequence Induction and Intubation: Current Controversy." *Anesthesia & Analgesia* 110, no. 5 (May 2010): 1318–1325.

Frerk, Chris, Viki S. Mitchell, Al F. McNarry, Cyprian Mendonca, Ravi Bhagrath, Anil Patel, Ellen P. O'Sullivan, Nicholas M. Woodall, and Imran Ahmad. Difficult Airway Society intubation guidelines working group. "Difficult Airway Society 2015 Guidelines for Management of Unanticipated Difficult Intubation in Adults." *British Journal of Anaesthesia* 115, no. 6 (December 2015): 1–22.

Sinclair, Rhona C. F., and Mark C. Luxton. "Rapid Sequence Induction." *Continuing Education in Anaesthesia, Critical Care & Pain* 5, no. 2 (April 2005):45–48.

Wallace, Claire, and Barry McGuire. "Rapid Sequence Induction: Its Place in Modern Anaesthesia." *Continuing Education in Anaesthesia, Critical Care & Pain* 14, no. 3 (June 2014): 1–6.

Weingart, Scott D., and Richard M. Levitan. "Preoxygenation and the Prevention of Desaturation During Emergency Airway Management." *Annals of Emergency Medicine* 59, no. 3 (March 2012): 165–175.

28

Endotracheal tube and tracheostomy problems

BRENDAN MCGRATH

'Quick! There's a problem at Bed 6!'

Critically ill patients can deteriorate suddenly for many reasons, but one of the most feared situations is an airway problem. Whatever the circumstances, a rapid but comprehensive assessment of the airway is always indicated.

Intubating a patient with an oral (or less commonly nasal) endotracheal tube can be difficult, but the majority of problems occur *after* intubation. The same is true for patients with a tracheostomy tube in situ. These artificial devices are prone to blockage (obstruction) or displacement.

WHEN DO AIRWAY PROBLEMS OCCUR?

High-risk periods include

- Initial intubation or during tracheostomy
- Patient movement for procedures or nursing care/rolls
- Sedation breaks or sedation reduction
- Transfers (e.g. to CT scanner)

Prompt assessment, recognition and action are required to prevent deterioration.

HOW WILL I KNOW IT IS AN AIRWAY PROBLEM?

Always consider this diagnosis in a distressed, tachypnoeic or hypoxic patient. Continuous monitoring should be in place for all invasively venti-lated patients. Waveform capnography is essential (see Figure 28.1). Changing or absent waveform can indicate a problem with

- The tube – usually blocked or displaced (the commonest cause by far)
- The 'circuit' – tubes and filters between the patient and the ventilator can get blocked with sputum or fluid
- The ventilator

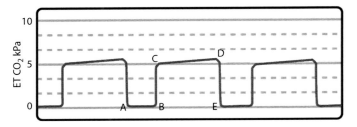

Figure 28.1 Capnography waveform.

- The patient's lungs – blockage in the major airways, severe bronchospasm or large pneumothorax
- The patient's circulation – the lungs need to be perfused to deliver CO_2 but a waveform will be present even with CPR

WHAT SHOULD I DO?

- Don't panic!
- Call for airway expert help.
    - Know who to call before you start your shift and how to get hold of them!
    - Remember senior ICU nurses will have seen these problems before.
- Give 100% oxygen.
- Oxygenation is the priority – you do not always need to give drugs or replace a tube straight away.
- Systematically troubleshoot, tackling the commonest problems first.

Most ICU nursing staff will have started to evaluate and manage the situation when you arrive. Clear communication is key. Removing the patient from the ventilator and connecting a new breathing circuit directly to the airway device eliminates potential problems with the existing circuit or ventilator. An 'Ambu bag' or 'Waters circuit' will usually be at the bedside.

SUSPECTED AIRWAY PROBLEM WITH THE ENDOTRACHEAL TUBE STILL IN THE MOUTH

An airway problem where the tube is partially displaced or obstructed can be difficult to diagnose, especially if the problem is visibly not obvious. Look, listen and feel for

- Changes in or absent waveform capnograph
- The patient biting the tube (may need a sedation bolus)
- Audible air leaking or gurgling from the mouth during ventilation
- Spontaneous attempts at breathing by the patient

ACTIONS

1. Call for expert help.
2. Disconnect the breathing circuit from the endotracheal tube.
3. IS THE TUBE IN THE AIRWAY?

   a. Look, listen and feel for spontaneous breathing at the mouth or end of the tube.
   b. Attempt to pass a suction catheter (ask the nurses for help).
   c. Attach an 'Ambu bag' or 'Waters circuit' and attempt gentle ventilation via the endotracheal tube with 100% oxygen (see Figure 28.2).
   d. Waveform capnography trace, clinical signs of ventilation (chest movement) and a suction catheter that easily passes indicate that the tube is in the airway. It may be partially blocked or displaced but ventilation is possible – do not remove but continue attempts at oxygenation/ventilation with 100% oxygen.
   e. Absence of these signs implies that the tube is completely displaced or blocked. Remove the tube and proceed as below.

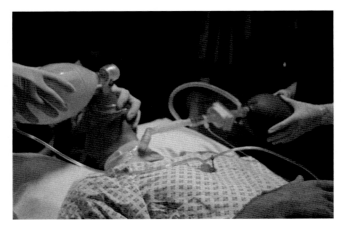

Figure 28.2 'Waters circuit' or 'Mapleson C circuit'. Spontaneous breathing can be monitored by observing bag movement and positive pressure can be applied by squeezing the bag. The adjustable pressure limit valve can control the pressure in the system.

WHAT TO DO IF THE ENDOTRACHEAL TUBE IS COMPLETELY DISPLACED

1. The diagnosis is usually visually obvious.
2. Call for expert help.
3. Open the airway and assess for breathing (see Chapter 27). Use capnography.
4. BREATHING.
    a. Keep airway open (may need adjuncts or suction).
    b. Apply oxygen via tight-fitting facemask.
    c. Consider non-invasive ventilation or manually supported spontaneous breathing if hypoxic.
    d. Continually reassess – the patient may stop breathing or need more invasive support (re-insertion of the endotracheal tube after sedation).
5. NOT BREATHING.
    a. Manual ventilation is required.
    b. Insertion of a second generation supraglottic airway device (SAD), such as an iGel or ProSeal™ LMA, is recommended if you know how to insert one.
    c. Face-mask ventilation (FMV) techniques (squeezing a bag) may work too but the seal is not as good and there is no protection against aspiration.
6. Hypoxic patients may lose cardiac output – check arterial line pressures and ECG. Start CPR as per standard Resus Council guidelines (www.resus.org.uk).
7. Improving oxygenation – wait for expert help for re-intubation decision and assistance.
8. Worsening oxygenation – see Difficult Airway Society (DAS) guidelines (www.das.uk.com).
    a. These guidelines permit three attempts at SAD placement or FMV with a different device (or operator) each time.
    b. There is no point persisting with a failed technique.
    c. Explain clearly to the assembled team what is happening.
    d. Re-intubation may be required. This could be difficult and the patient may be haemodynamically unstable.
    e. Cannot intubate, cannot ventilate scenarios will require emergency front-of-neck airway (FONA). DAS guidelines suggest a scalpel-bougie cricothyroidotomy.

TRACHEOSTOMY BASICS

A tracheotomy is an artificial opening that has been surgically (or percutaneously) formed in the anterior trachea, which allows a stoma to be created from the skin of the anterior neck to the trachea – the tracheostomy. Tubes may be inserted through this stoma to allow the following:

- Continued ventilation
- A cuff to be inflated in order to
  - 'Seal off' the pharynx and upper airway (reducing the risk of aspiration)
  - Allow positive pressure to be administered
- Suctioning and 'airway toilet' to be performed without traumatising the soft tissues

Tracheostomy tubes are described in terms of the following characteristics:

- Their internal diameter and length (some are adjustable to allow their use in patients with larger necks).
- The presence of a cuff. It is not possible to ventilate the lungs effectively through an uncuffed tracheostomy or a cuffed tracheostomy with a deflated cuff.
- The presence of an inner removable cannula, which reduces the risk of the tube becoming blocked with secretions.
- The presence of a 'fenestration' or hole in the tube to allow air to move upwards through the larynx, which can allow the patient to talk. It is not possible to effectively ventilate the lungs through a fenestrated tube.

SURGICAL TRACHEOSTOMIES

- The anterior portions of two tracheal rings are removed.
- The stoma may be stitched open and the 'stay sutures' brought up to the skin surface to aid tube re-insertion.
- Easier to re-insert than percutaneous tracheostomies, especially after 3–4 days post-procedure.

PERCUTANEOUS TRACHEOSTOMIES

- Insertion involves a dilatational Seldinger wire technique.
- More difficult to re-insert before 7–10 days post-procedure.

Laryngectomy patients

During a laryngectomy, the larynx is removed and the trachea is stitched to the anterior neck. These patients have no communication between the oral/nasal cavities and the trachea/lungs, so they cannot be oxygenated or ventilated via the nose or mouth. In these patients, oxygen must be applied to the tracheal stoma, and any attempts at ventilation must occur via this stoma.

Mini-tracheostomy

This is usually inserted through the cricothyroid membrane to allow suctioning of secretions. It can be used to 'downsize' a tracheostomy stoma when a tracheostomy tube is removed, either to keep a tract open (if the tracheostomy might need to be re-inserted) or to provide help with secretion management when ventilation is no longer required. The lack of a cuff and the narrow lumen preclude its use for mechanical ventilation, although oxygen can be administered if necessary.

MANAGING TRACHEOSTOMY EMERGENCIES

Tracheostomy patients may present with worrying or red flag signs. These may herald a sudden deterioration and require urgent review by an experienced doctor. Red flags include the following:

- A suction catheter not passing easily into the trachea
- A changing, inadequate or absent capnograph trace
- Increasing ventilator support or increasing oxygen requirements
- Respiratory distress
- The patient suddenly being able to talk, or 'bubbling' of secretions in the mouth (indicating that gas is escaping proximally and the cuff is no longer 'sealing' the trachea)
- Frequent requirement for (excessive) inflation of the cuff to prevent air leak
- Pain at the tracheostomy site
- Surgical (subcutaneous) emphysema (gas in the soft tissues)
- Suspicion of aspiration (feed aspirated on tracheal toilet, which suggests that the cuff is not functioning adequately)

Two algorithms for the management of the tracheostomy patient with breathing difficulties are presented on pages 216 and 217. It is important to distinguish patients with a patent upper airway from those without one (laryngectomy patients).

- Oxygen should be applied to both the face and stoma.
- Anaesthetics/critical care and ENT/maxillofacial surgery should be called urgently, and a bronchoscope should be requested.
- A key step is to decide whether the patient's respiratory distress is due to blockage, displacement or some other cause (e.g. pneumothorax).
- Look, listen and feel for breath at the tube end, look for movement of a Water's circuit when attached to the tracheostomy, look for a capnograph trace, and look at the patient's chest.
- If an inner tube is present, it should be removed, unblocked and replaced.
- Reassess breathing at the mouth/nose and the tracheostomy.
- If the patient is not breathing and the tracheostomy is not patent (a suction catheter will not pass), vigorous attempts at ventilation may make the situation worse by causing surgical emphysema.
- Try deflating the cuff as the patient may be able to breathe around a blocked or displaced tube – reassess.
- If this does not result in improvement, the tracheostomy should be removed (unless an airway expert is present and safe adequate oxygenation is occurring via the facial route, in which case the tracheostomy may be manipulated).
- The patient may now require orotracheal intubation, re-intubation of the stoma, or the use of other airway adjuncts (e.g. laryngeal mask airway). The decision as to which is the most appropriate will depend upon the following:
  - The anticipated difficulty of orotracheal intubation
  - Whether a tract is well formed (at least 72 hours for a surgical tracheostomy and 7–10 days for a percutaneous one)
  - The doctor's skills
  - Clinical urgency
- The goal is a stable, oxygenated patient. If you do not have the skills to safely insert a tracheostomy tube or an endotracheal tube, and the patient is stable, wait for an expert.

EXPERT TIPS

- An LMA or paediatric face-mask applied to the stoma can be an effective seal and allow ventilation without a tracheostomy tube.
- Sedating a spontaneously breathing, stable patient can be dangerous if they have a difficult upper airway and tracheostomy. This should only be done if the right skills, equipment and personnel are available, and it may require a trip to theatre in order to be done safely.
- An Aintree catheter loaded onto a fibre-optic bronchoscope is much better than trying to poke a bougie or similar instrument into a precarious stoma.

So, when somebody shouts 'Quick! There's a problem at Bed 6!'...

- Rapid, comprehensive assessment of the airway.
- Oxygenation is the priority.
- Call for expert help.
- Start with the basics and use more invasive techniques as the situation and your training allow.
- If the airway is patent, move on to the rest of ABCDE assessment.

FURTHER READING

Difficult Airway Society. "Difficult Airway Society." www.das.uk.com (accessed 21 January 2017).

McGrath, Brendan A., Lucy Bates, Dougal Atkinson, and John A. Moore. "Multidisciplinary Guidelines for the Management of Tracheostomy and Laryngectomy Airway Emergencies." *Anaesthesia* 67, no. 9 (June 2012): 1025–1041.

National Tracheostomy Safety Project. "NTSP - UK National Tracheostomy Safety Project Home." www.tracheostomy.org.uk/ (accessed 21 January 2017).

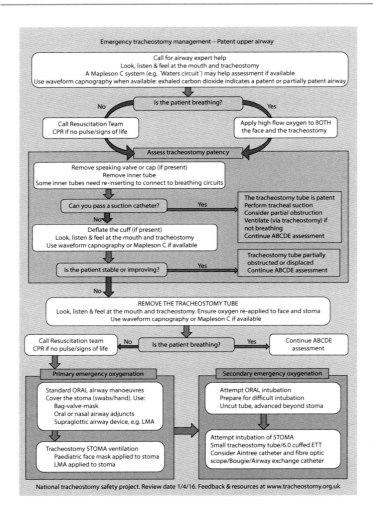

Emergency tracheostomy management – Patent upper airway

Call for airway expert help
Look, listen & feel at the mouth and tracheostomy
A Mapleson C system (e.g. 'Waters circuit') may help assessment if available
Use waveform capnography when available: exhaled carbon dioxide indicates a patent or partially patent airway

Is the patient breathing?

No

Yes

Call Resuscitation Team
CPR if no pulse/signs of life

Apply high flow oxygen to BOTH
the face and the tracheostomy

Assess tracheostomy patency

Remove speaking valve or cap (if present)
Remove inner tube
Some inner tubes need re-inserting to connect to breathing circuits

Can you pass a suction catheter?   Yes

No

The tracheostomy tube is patent
Perform tracheal suction
Consider partial obstruction
Ventilate (via tracheostomy) if
not breathing
Continue ABCDE assessment

Deflate the cuff (if present)
Look, listen & feel at the mouth and tracheostomy
Use waveform capnography or Mapleson C if available

Is the patient stable or improving?   Yes

Tracheostomy tube partially
obstructed or displaced
Continue ABCDE assessment

No

REMOVE THE TRACHEOSTOMY TUBE
Look, listen & feel at the mouth and tracheostomy. Ensure oxygen re-applied to face and stoma
Use waveform capnography or Mapleson C if available

Call Resuscitation team
CPR if no pulse/signs of life   No   Is the patient breathing?   Yes   Continue ABCDE
assessment

Primary emergency oxygenation

Secondary emergency oxygenation

Standard ORAL airway manoeuvres
Cover the stoma (swabs/hand). Use:
Bag-valve-mask
Oral or nasal airway adjuncts
Supraglottic airway device, e.g. LMA

Attempt ORAL intubation
Prepare for difficult intubation
Uncut tube, advanced beyond stoma

Attempt intubation of STOMA
Small tracheostomy tube/6.0 cuffed ETT
Consider Aintree catheter and fibre optic
scope/Bougie/Airway exchange catheter

Tracheostomy STOMA ventilation
Paediatric face mask applied to stoma
LMA applied to stoma

National tracheostomy safety project. Review date 1/4/16. Feedback & resources at www.tracheostomy.org.uk

Algorithm 28.1

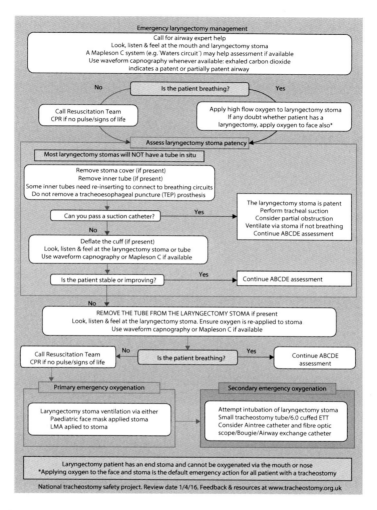

Algorithm 28.2

'The Association of Anaesthetists of Great Britain & Ireland grants readers the right to reproduce the algorithms included in this article (Algorithms 28.1 and 28.2) for non-commercial purposes (including in scholarly journals, books and

29

'Fighting the ventilator'

MOHAMMED HATAB AND PETER FRANK

'I can't ventilate my patient – could you come and review him?'

A 26-year-old male was admitted to the intensive care following a road traffic collision. The patient required intubation and ventilation on arrival due to agitation and hypoxia. A CT scan was performed revealing bilateral lung contusions, fractures of the second and third ribs on the right side, but no pneumothorax. After 48 hours of uneventful mechanical ventilation, the patient begins to need higher airway pressures, and his oxygen requirement is increasing. The nursing staff reports that he is starting to 'fight the ventilator'.

QUESTIONS

1. What are the likely causes for a patient to start fighting mechanical ventilation in this setting?
2. What would be the next steps in your management of this patient?
3. What further investigations might be required?

INTRODUCTION

The term 'fighting the ventilator' is used to describe the situation where a mechanically ventilated patient is showing signs of agitation, with or without evidence of respiratory distress. This can happen when a patient becomes agitated, sedation levels fall or they try to breathe against the ventilator, also known as dyssynchrony. Each of these problems will cause a rise in airway pressure and ultimately a fall in minute volume, leading to hypoxia and hypercarbia. Without prompt treatment, both respiratory and cardiovascular collapse can occur, making ventilator dyssynchrony an important issue that requires urgent appropriate intervention.

INITIAL ASSESSMENT

An immediate decision about the severity of the problem should be made. Hypoxia and hypercarbia are emergency situations and should be dealt with in a structured 'ABC' manner as described below. When respiratory failure is occurring, the most useful initial step is often to remove the ventilator completely by attaching a Water's circuit and ventilating with 100% oxygen. This will often improve oxygenation and allow you the time to perform the following assessment:

- Call for help.
- A: Check the position of the endotracheal (ET) tube, and ensure that there are no kinks or blockages.
- B: Assess adequacy of ventilation. Can you hear breath sounds bilaterally? Is chest expansion adequate? Are there any added sounds such as wheeze or crepitations?
- C: Check whether blood pressure and heart rate are haemodynamically stable.

IDENTIFICATION OF THE PROBLEM

If the patient is stable and there is no emergency treatment required, or once the patient has been successfully resuscitated, troubleshooting to identify the cause of dyssynchrony can commence. This can be divided into the following four broad areas.

AIRWAY OR BREATHING CIRCUIT ISSUES

- ET tube. Is it blocked (due to kinks or secretions)? Has it travelled into the right main bronchus?
- Circuit. Is the circuit kinked? Are there any pools of fluid causing increased resistance? Check for disconnections.

BREATHING OR CIRCULATORY PROBLEMS

- LOOK for chest movement, tracheal deviation and asymmetry of ventilation.
- FEEL for hyperresonance, tracheal deviation, surgical emphysema (suggesting a pneumothorax) and dullness in-keeping with pleural effusions/collapse.
- LISTEN for adequacy of air entry, and added sounds such as crepitations in pulmonary oedema/consolidation/ARDS, wheeze and reduced air entry in severe bronchospasm, etc.
- Assess for circulatory collapse, which could be accounting for respiratory distress.

INAPPROPRIATE VENTILATOR SETTINGS

- A fully mandatory mode or a mode without any pressure support is being used for a patient who is trying to make spontaneous breaths. This can be uncomfortable and difficult for a lightly sedated patient to tolerate. Switching to a mode that allows supported spontaneous breaths will usually solve this issue.
- The trigger is not sensitive enough; the patient wants to trigger but cannot generate sufficient inspiratory flow or pressure for the ventilator to sense their attempt to breathe. Reducing the flow trigger to approximately 1 L/min should help to overcome this.

- Flow rate is inadequate to meet inspiratory flow demand. This can make a patient feel like they have to work harder to take a full breath, resulting in a gasping or 'air hunger' appearance. Increasing the flow rate or altering the shape of the pressure time curve by adjusting the 'ramp' settings may alleviate this.
- Gas trapping within the patient's chest. In situations where expiratory flow may be prolonged, there may be insufficient time for full exhalation to occur. This can result in gas accumulating in the chest resulting in a rise in intrathoracic pressure during expiration known as 'auto-PEEP'. When this occurs, the lungs may be operating at the top of their compliance curve, with the result that the patient has to work hard to increase their volume and draw more gas in. Providing extrinsic PEEP may alleviate this, but it may exacerbate it too. Therefore, once gas trapping has been identified, expert advice is required.

INADEQUATE SEDATION OR PARALYSIS

- Is the patient appropriately sedated? Simply increasing the sedation level may help the patient to tolerate the ventilator.
- Assess for other causes of discomfort or agitation. Any degree of pain can cause a patient to 'fight' the ventilator. For example, they may have a full bladder or bowel that is causing considerable discomfort, or if the patient has had surgery, has adequate analgesia been provided?
- Some patients requiring high levels of ventilator support may need muscle relaxants to allow ventilation, even if adequately sedated (e.g. ARDS patients). The decision to paralyse a patient to facilitate ventilation should be made by an experienced intensivist to avoid the situation where a patient may be aware but paralysed.

CONCLUSION

- Dyssynchrony may result because of factors that are related to the patient or that are related to the ventilator settings or a problem with the endotracheal tube, tracheostomy tube or the circuit. The main aim is to stabilize the patient and once there is good ventilation and oxygenation, you can troubleshoot the problem.

- Patient-ventilator dyssynchrony can prolong mechanical ventilation and hospital stay.
- Sedation is a common solution for managing dyssynchrony, but it may not always be the best answer for all types of dyssynchrony.
- Optimising ventilation for patients who are requiring a mixture of mandatory and supported breaths is complex, and requires a full understanding of both respiratory physiology and ventilator operating characteristics.

KEY LEARNING POINTS

- Patients not synchronising with ventilation, or 'fighting the ventilator', are common and are a significant cause for concern.
- Identification of the underlying reason for the dyssynchrony requires a systematic approach and is key to solving the problem.
- In challenging cases or in an emergency, manually ventilating the patient can help identify whether the problem is mainly patient related, or due to incorrect ventilator settings.

FURTHER READING

Bersten, Andrew D. *Oh's Intensive Care Manual*. 7th ed. Oxford: Butterworth-Heinemann Elsevier, 2013.

Gilstrap, Daniel, and Neil MacIntyre. "Patient–Ventilator Interactions: Implications for Clinical Management." *American Journal of Respiratory and Critical Care Medicine* 188, no. 9 (November 2013): 1058–1068.

Topin, Martin J. *Principles and Practice of Mechanical Ventilation*. 3rd ed. New York: McGraw-Hill Book Company, 2013.

30

Pneumothorax

GARETH P. JONES AND AMANDA SHAW

A young man in his early twenties is admitted following a car accident. He is currently intubated and invasively ventilated. You are called to see him because his saturations are falling but as you arrive, you notice that one side of his chest is not moving. The tube placement has been confirmed on a chest film and the nurse is ventilating with a bag and valve. There is no obstruction to the tube on suction. What do you need to do?

Pneumothorax is a common cause of breathlessness in critical care patients, especially following trauma.

DEFINITION

A pneumothorax is the term for a collection of air around the lungs, between the lungs and chest wall (i.e. between the visceral and parietal pleura).

CAUSES

Essentially due to a tear in the lung that allows air to escape and collect in the pleural space. They can be termed *primary* or *secondary* depending on whether they are related to an underlying lung disease. They can be spontaneous or due to another cause, e.g. trauma:

1. *Spontaneous*
   a. *Primary*
      i. No apparent cause
      ii. Occurring mainly in healthy young people – especially tall and thin young men
   b. *Secondary*
      i. As a result of an underlying condition, e.g. bullae in COPD. Those over 50 who smoke are considered to have secondary pneumothorax.
2. *Traumatic*
   As a result of direct trauma to the chest (could be external, e.g. chest injury, or internal, e.g. ventilator over inflation. Could also be deliberate, e.g. during chest surgery).

RECOGNITION

Depending on the size of the pneumothorax and the state of the patient, the *symptoms* may be absent to severe:

- Sharp chest pain worse on inspiration
- Shortness of breath
- Wheeze

Signs can include the following:

- Hypoxia – may present as low peripheral oxygen saturations or low PaO_2 on an arterial blood gas sample
- Cyanosis (blue tinge around the lips and tongue)

- Tachypnoea (rapid breathing)
- Tachycardia (increased heart rate)
- Rising ventilation pressures with no clear reason

If there is building pressure in the chest, this can displace the mediastinum and is termed a *tension pneumothorax* (see section on page 228). This may cause the following:

- Hypotension (low blood pressure)
- Distended neck veins
- Rise in CVP (central venous pressure) (normal ≤12 mmHg)
- Tracheal deviation (away from the side of the pneumothorax)
- Ventilated patients may appear to 'fight' the ventilator

(If tension pneumothorax is identified, you must act immediately! Insert a large-bore cannula into the second intercostal space in the midclavicular line of the affected side.)

Good *examination* is key to the early recognition of pneumothorax, as there may not be time for a chest radiograph for confirmation!

Inspection – One side of the chest may not be moving as well and tracheal deviation may be visible.

Palpation – Again, chest expansion may be reduced on palpation. The cardiac apex may also be displaced.

Percussion – The chest may be hyperresonant over the pneumothorax (like a drum).

Auscultation – There may be decreased or even absent breath sounds over the pneumothorax.

A plain chest radiograph is often useful in identifying pneumothorax. However, as mentioned above, if the patient is unwell, it may be necessary to treat before a radiograph is available. For a diagnosis on a radiograph, there must be two features present:

1. Visible lung edge
2. Absence of lung markings lateral to the lung edge

TIP

Pneumothoraces are often overlooked in the apex, especially where the lung edge may follow the contour of a rib.

TENSION PNEUMOTHORAX

This refers to a condition where the pressure of the air in the pneumothorax has built sufficiently to press the mediastinum (centre of the chest) over. This is a life-threatening condition and must be treated immediately.

Tension pneumothorax is more common in patients who are mechanically ventilated. This is because the ventilator is pushing air into the lungs, whereas, in a spontaneously breathing patient, the air is sucked in. The 'tear' in the lung tissue acts as a valve allowing the pressure to build. Therefore, pneumothorax in a ventilated patient may lead to *rapid deterioration. If prompt action is not taken, the patient may die.*

MANAGEMENT – WHAT DO YOU NEED TO DO?

1. If you are not experienced in managing pneumothorax, call for experienced help.
2. Give the patient high-flow oxygen (10–15 L/min via a non-rebreathe mask) OR increase the oxygen to 100% in ventilated patients.

In a patient who is not mechanically ventilated:

- *Small pneumothorax* (<2 cm rim of air on the chest radiograph and not causing breathlessness): monitoring. In a primary pneumothorax, discharge can be considered with outpatient follow up in 2–4 weeks. Secondary pneumothoraces should be monitored as an inpatient for at least 24 hours.
- *Larger pneumothorax* (>2 cm or breathless): aspiration should be attempted with a 16–18 g cannula. If this resolves the pneumothorax, the patient may only require further monitoring. If it does not resolve it, a 12–14 Fr ((Fr)ench gauge is three times the diameter in millimetres) chest drain should be inserted.
- *Tension pneumothorax* is an emergency and requires prompt action. Insert a large-bore cannula (14 g) in the second intercostal space in the midclavicular line. A chest drain will then be required.

In patients who are mechanically ventilated, a chest drain is usually required; however, as mentioned above, they are also at much higher risk of tension pneumothorax:

- *Pneumothorax* in a ventilated patient: insert an intercostal chest drain.

- *Tension pneumothorax*: insert a large bore cannula (14 g) in the second intercostal space in the midclavicular line. A chest drain will then be required.

CHEST DRAIN INSERTION

There are two techniques commonly used in the insertion of a chest drain and the choice depends on the operator, the patient and the size of the pneumothorax.

1. *Seldinger chest drain* – This technique is used in a variety of drains and lines including arterial lines, central lines and ascetic drains and the technique remains the same. This is commonly employed as a first line chest drain, especially in medical specialities.
2. *'Surgical' chest drain* – A larger bore tube is inserted after blunt dissection through the thoracic cage. These are often employed second line, following thoracic surgery, e.g. cardio-oesophagectomy and in larger pneumothoraces requiring aggressive drainage.

TECHNIQUE

1. Place the patient as comfortably as possible in a supine or semi-recumbent position with the affected side slightly elevated. You should also consider the patient's position in relation to yourself so that you are comfortable as you could be there for some time.
2. Consider premedication with analgesia and/or an anxiolytic as appropriate. It is a painful procedure!
3. Flex the patient's arm over their head or on the hip to improve access to the area.
4. Clean the chest wall (e.g. with a chlorhexidine- or iodine-based wash) and cover with sterile drapes (if there is time).
5. Put on a surgical cap and mask, scrub your hands and put on a gown and sterile gloves (again if there is time).
6. Instil local anaesthetic into the chosen site (usually the fifth intercostal space, anterior axillary line).
7. The drain can then be inserted either with a Seldinger technique or surgical technique – aiming for the apex (top) of the chest wall.

8. The drain should be secured with a suture.
9. Connect the drain to a bottle with an underwater seal – there are usually special bottles designed for this purpose. Bubbles should appear in the water if it is working.
10. Apply sterile dressings to the area of the chest drain.
11. Check the position of the drain with a chest radiograph.
12. The patient should then be closely monitored for changes, which may include further chest radiographs to assess changes in the pneumothorax.

FURTHER READING

Havelock, Tom, Richard Teoh, Diane Laws, and Fergus Gleeson. "Pleural Procedures and Thoracic Ultrasound: British Thoracic Society Pleural Disease Guideline 2010." *Thorax* 65, Supplement 2 (2010): 61–76.

Hinds, Charles J., and David Watson. *Intensive Care: a Concise Textbook*. 3rd ed. Philadelphia, PA: Saunders Elsevier, 2008, pp. 165–166.

MacDuff, Andrew, Anthony Arnold, and John Harvey. "Management of Spontaneous Pneumothorax: British Thoracic Society Pleural Disease Guideline 2010." *Thorax* 5, Supplement 2 (2010): 18–31.

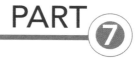

PART 7

OTHER EMERGENCIES

31

Cardiac arrhythmias

KATHERINE TURNER, PETER BUNTING AND MIKE DICKINSON

'The patient in Bed 8 has a heart rate of 150. Please can you come and have a look?'

Cardiac arrhythmias are common in sick patients in Critical Care and this is a very common scenario.

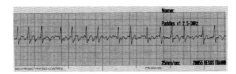

Figure 31.1 Normal sinus rhythm.

Arrhythmias can be classified according to their origin, as supraventricular or ventricular, or their effect on heart rate, as bradycardias or tachycardias. The effect that arrhythmia has on the cardiac output and blood pressure determines whether or not it is life threatening. Management depends on the type of arrhythmia; some arrhythmias are cardiac arrest rhythms and require immediate treatment following the Advanced Life Support (ALS) principles of airway, breathing and circulation.

The first step is to recognise the abnormal rhythm. Figure 31.1 illustrates normal sinus rhythm, with each P wave followed by a QRS complex and a T wave.

SUPRAVENTRICULAR ARRHYTHMIAS

SUPRAVENTRICULAR TACHYCARDIA (SVT)

Supraventricular tachycardias can be divided into regular or irregular rhythms.

- Regular: initiated from the sinoatrial (SA) node as sinus tachycardias
- Irregular: initiated by un-coordinated contraction of the atrial muscle (atrial fibrillation)

ATRIAL FIBRILLATION

Atrial fibrillation (AF) is the most common arrhythmia in critical care (Figure 31.2) and one that you will often be asked to review. The rhythm is irregularly irregular, and if there is an arterial line in place, the height and width of each arterial pulse will vary.

AF is commonly associated with the following:

- Hypovolaemia
- Electrolyte disturbances (most commonly low potassium and low magnesium levels)

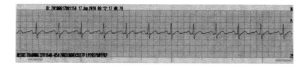

Figure 31.2 Atrial fibrillation.

- Acid–base abnormalities
- Cardiac ischaemia
- Valvular heart disease
- Inflammatory processes (e.g. middle lobe pneumonia causing irritation of the atrial muscle)

Cardiac output may not be compromised in slow AF, but if the rate is fast, the cardiac output may be reduced.

TREATMENT

1. Electrocardiography – should be performed for every patient.
2. Bloods (electrolytes, blood gases and acid–base status) – myocardial cells cannot function properly in acidic or hypoxic environments.
3. Measure preload (volume status) – correct if abnormal to enable normal atrial function.
4. Drugs – if the patient has a good cardiac output and stable blood pressure, then consider drug therapy; amiodarone is first-line. Digoxin or beta-blockers may be used for rate control.
5. Direct-current (DC) cardioversion – if the patient's blood pressure is compromised and cardiac output is life threatening.

ATRIAL TACHYCARDIA

In some circumstances, atrial tachycardia can be physiological; during exercise the heart rate can approach 180 beats/min, but in the ICU, it is always pathological. On an ECG, you will see narrow complex tachycardias (Figure 31.3).

TREATMENT

1. Adenosine – will stop the action potential of the AV node and cause a few seconds of ventricular standstill, the heart then resuming in normal sinus rhythm. If the rhythm is AF or atrial flutter, the heart will not revert to normal sinus rhythm, as these rhythms are independent of the AV node.

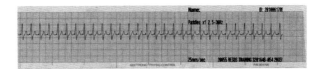

Figure 31.3 Atrial tachycardia.

SUPRAVENTRICULAR BRADYCARDIAS

The SA node can be ischaemic, and any critical illness can cause critical ischaemia and failure of the node. The result may be a sick sinus syndrome or failure to initiate the normal rhythm and a bradycardia.

HEART BLOCK

These rhythm abnormalities are due to the propagated action potential in the heart being prevented from progressing down the normal pathway.

They can be classified as follows:

1. *First-degree*
   Usually benign in isolation but capable of progressing to higher degrees of block if provoked by drugs that decrease the activity of excitable tissue, such as anaesthetic, sedative agents and beta-blockers.
2. *Second-degree* (subdivided into Mobitz I or Wenkebach and Mobitz II)
   Can cause a drop in blood pressure because of missed beats, and like first-degree heart block can progress.
3. *Third-degree*
   There is complete disassociation between atrial and ventricular activity. The cells of the AV node act as a pacemaker for the ventricles. The inherent rate of these cells is approximately 40 beats per minute. In most patients, there will be a drop in cardiac output of about 50%, which will be symptomatic (Figures 31.4 through 31.7).

TREATMENT

There are currently no drug treatments available for heart block; the only treatment option is electrical pacing. The electrical signal is blocked from progressing through the normal pathway, so external electricity is used to cause contraction of the ventricle. Treatment depends on whether the patient

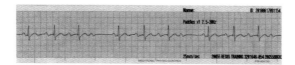

Figure 31.4 First-degree heart block.

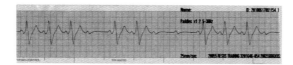

Figure 31.5 Second-degree heart block (Mobitz Type I).

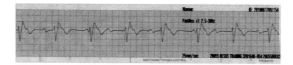

Figure 31.6 Second-degree heart block (Mobitz Type II).

Figure 31.7 Third-degree heart block.

is symptomatic or not. In a symptomatic patient, external pacing pads should be used. If the patient is asymptomatic, or is stable, transvenous pacing can be used.

VENTRICULAR ARRHYTHMIAS

VENTRICULAR EXTRASYSTOLES

Ventricular extrasystoles (Figure 31.8) are common and are of no consequence if they are infrequent. If they are frequent (i.e. 1 in 2 or 3 beats), they

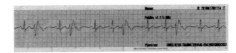

Figure 31.8 Ventricular extrasystoles.

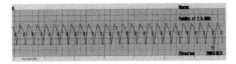

Figure 31.9 Ventricular tachycardia.

may cause a fall in cardiac output. Ventricular tachycardia is a run of extrasystoles (Figure 31.9); it can be slow, but is usually fast, at least 120 beats per minute. The cardiac output may be preserved or compromised.

TREATMENT

1. Urgent DC cardioversion is the most effective treatment.
2. Drugs – may be used to stabilise membranes.

VENTRICULAR FIBRILLATION

Ventricular fibrillation may be coarse or fine but is always a cardiac arrest rhythm and requires urgent resuscitation. Whilst preparing the defibrillator, the ALS principles of airway, breathing and circulation should be followed to ensure the myocardium is not hypoxic and acidotic. Good CPR should ensure some blood flow to and maintenance of the function of vital organs (Figures 31.10 and 31.11).

ASYSTOLE

Figure 31.12 shows asystole. Asystole is always a cardiac arrest rhythm and CPR should be started as per the ALS protocol.

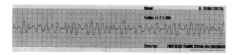

Figure 31.10 Coarse ventricular fibrillation.

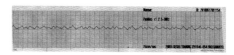

Figure 31.11 Fine ventricular fibrillation.

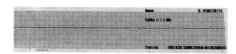

Figure 31.12 Asystole.

KEY LEARNING POINTS

- Cardiac arrhythmias are common in sick patients in critical care and have varying implications.
- Arrhythmias can be classified according to origin or their effect on heart rate.
- The most common arrhythmia is atrial fibrillation.

32

ICU delirium and the agitated patient

NICHOLAS R. PLUMMER AND SHONDIPON K. LAHA

'Mr Smith is pulling at his lines and is distressed tonight. Can you prescribe something to sedate him?'

WHAT IS CRITICAL CARE DELIRIUM?

Delirium is common in critical care patients, with many considering it an ubiquitous feature of critical illness. Critical care delirium is a sudden, fluctuating disturbance in attention with altered levels of arousal and cognition, which occurs with physical or mental illness. It is characterised by the cardinal feature of inattention (reduced ability to direct, focus, sustain and shift attention) alongside an altered level of consciousness, difficulties in processing normal thoughts and disruption to sleep–wake cycles.

CAUSES AND IMPACT OF CRITICAL CARE DELIRIUM AND AGITATION

Delirium affects 16%–89% of patients in intensive care. Risk factors include increasing age, the presence of more than one condition associated with altered level of consciousness or coma, treatment with sedative agents, new neurological diagnoses or insults, pre-existing medical and psychiatric comorbidities, metabolic abnormalities, withdrawal from chronic psychoactive substances (including alcohol and nicotine), sleep deprivation, elevated ambient noise and increased severity of illness.

The pathophysiology of critical care delirium is multi-factorial, largely uncharacterised, and poorly understood. In addition to an association with sedative agents, there are potential links with the use of GABA-agonists, anticholinergics, beta-blockers and digoxin. Some suggest delirium is associated with excess dopaminergic activity (similar to psychosis and schizophrenia), and there is likely a direct neurotoxic effect of inflammatory cytokines in sepsis and post-surgery.

Clinically, delirium appears to interplay with the other two aspects of the 'ICU triad': pain and psychological agitation. Delirium is worsened by anxiety and frustration (be this appropriate to the patient's clinical condition or pathological), lack of physiological homeostasis (e.g. thirst, hunger or dyspnoea during respiratory weaning), and inability to communicate. Additional concerns and anxieties arise in the setting of intensive care, in particular lack of orientation to time and space, and separation from relatives. Painful procedures – anything from the presence of endotracheal tubes through to tissue injury, as well as routine elements of ICU care, such as vascular access, turning and physiotherapy – further interact with delirium and agitation, with patients ascribing this a profound unpleasant affective component ('this pain means I'm more likely to die'), which further worsens their psychological state.

Delirium is not only disturbing and de-humanising for patients, but is associated with increased duration of mechanical ventilation, longer critical care and hospital lengths of stay, increased all-cause mortality (10% increase in relative risk of death with each day of delirium), and long-term cognitive impairment and reduced functional status on discharge. Agitation and delirium increase nursing burden, and the risk of the patient injuring themselves or dislodging lines and airway devices. Delirium is also distressing for patient's relatives, and features significantly in the memory of ICU survivors, even if they lacked insight into their delirium at the time. Functional imaging has demonstrated cerebral atrophy and white-matter disruption associated with increased duration of delirium. Early detection and intervention is important, as the longer the duration of delirium, the worse the associated outcomes and the harder it becomes to treat.

DETECTING DELIRIUM

To be able to manage delirium, we need to identify it. Unfortunately, delirium is commonly misdiagnosed, or just missed entirely. The clinical impression of both nurses and doctors has been shown to be a poor assessment, especially if the patient is not hyperactive, with staff missing over 75% of cases based on clinical assessment alone.

Clinically, critical care delirium takes one of three forms:

- **Hypoactive delirium**
  Inattention, disordered thinking and decreased level of consciousness without agitation
- **Hyperactive delirium**
  Similar to hypoactive delirium, but with agitation
- **Mixed delirium**

Although floridly hyperactive patients are the easiest to recognise, pure hyperactive delirium accounts for less than 2% of all cases. Patients are far more likely to experience hypoactive delirium, which also has a higher associated mortality; however, survivors have better long-term cognitive outcomes than those with hyperactive or mixed delirium.

The Diagnostic and Statistical Manual of Mental Disorders, 5th edition (DSM-V) gives four criteria for the diagnosis of delirium:

- *Disturbance in attention* (i.e. reduced ability to direct, focus, sustain and shift attention) and awareness.
- *Change in cognition* (e.g. memory deficit, disorientation, language disturbance, perceptual disturbance) that is not better accounted for by established or evolving dementia.
- *Develops over a short period* (hours to days) and tends to fluctuate during the course of the day.

- *Evidence* from history, examination or investigations that the disturbance is caused by a direct consequence of a medical condition, an intoxicating substance, medication use or combinations of the above causes.

It is interesting to note that light sedation – to which many critical care patients are exposed – can fulfil all of the DSM-V criteria for delirium, and that there is a significant overlap between the features of delirium, signs of agitation, and the physiological and psychological response to pain. Therefore, we need tools to enable us to apply these DSM criteria to critically ill patients with rapidly fluctuating severity of illness, who are receiving multiple analgesic and sedative agents, and who often cannot speak due to airway devices or pathology.

Any such tools must be used in concert with a sedation scale, as this will allow us to distinguish between the impact of sedative drugs and pathological delirium, and hypoactive and hyperactive states. The Richmond Agitation-Sedation Scale (RASS) is used in many critical care units for this purpose. Patients are scored from –5 to +4, with negative scores indicating deeper sedation and positive scores agitation; 0 is the appearance of calm, normal alertness. If RASS ≥–3 (moderate sedation), the patient should then be screened for delirium.

Multiple tools exist for assessing the presence of delirium, including the Confusion Assessment Method for ICU (CAM-ICU), the Intensive Care Delirium Screening Checklist (ICDSC), the opinion of a treating doctor or nurse, or formal cognitive testing by a geriatrician or psychiatrist. There are also numerous challenges to bedside testing for delirium, in particular muscle weakness or restricted movement, the inability to vocalise, sensory impairment, and patients who deliberately give alternative answers – patients in follow up clinic have said that they knew they were delirious, yet gave negative answers as they did not want to be treated!

The most commonly used screening tool is CAM-ICU, a two-step system that first assesses level of consciousness using RASS, and then assesses for confusion and inattention. It is well validated and highly specific, although recent studies have shown that it can be more poorly sensitive than first thought when used pragmatically by nursing staff, in particular under-reporting hypoactive delirium. Its main limitations are that it relies on a subjective change from baseline, issues a binary outcome rather than a likelihood of delirium or assessment of severity, is assessed only at a single point in time (although a positive result should trigger further assessments at twelve hourly intervals), and does not consider the impact of sedation aside from in ensuring that the patient is not too heavily sedated to be screenable (Figure 32.1).

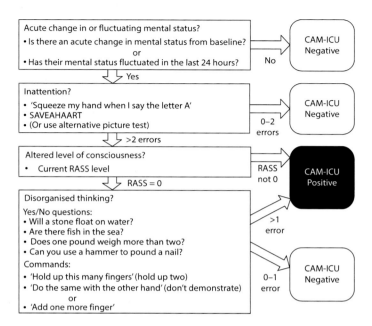

Figure 32.1 CAM-ICU screening flowchart.

Alternatives to CAM-ICU include the ICDSC, which can be thought of more as an assessment of 'fragility' to delirium over time rather than simply assessing presence or severity; research tools that aim to detect attention deficits, such as the EDTB-ICU attention score (an objective test run using an electronic device) and DELAPP-ICU (a smartphone app that assesses behaviour, then runs a sustained attention task), or physiological methods including eye moments, heart rate variability, temperature variability and EEG signal. However, none have yet been as well validated or are as straightforward to use as CAM-ICU.

MANAGEMENT OF CRITICAL CARE DELIRIUM AND AGITATION

All patients in critical care are at risk of delirium, and although it is not entirely preventable, some general measures should be put in place to reduce the risk and severity of delirium affecting any ICU patient. A high index of suspicion for delirium must be maintained, and patients screened at least every twelve hours by nursing staff and during daily reviews by medical staff.

A general strategy involves minimising sedation, including regular use of sedation holds and targeting sedation so that patients tolerate treatment, but are no more sedated than this. Higher sedation levels have been retrospectively linked with increased delirium rates and higher all-cause ICU mortality, and sedative agents (especially propofol and benzodiazepines) are well known to disrupt sleep architecture. Their impact is worsened by the addition of cytochrome P450 inhibitors, which particularly worsen delirium secondary to midazolam and fentanyl. Practically, this involves prescribing sedation to a RASS target, and using 'analgesia-first' regimes, aiming to control pain and keep patients comfortable rather than use large doses of sedative agents.

Management of pain in ICU can be difficult, as patients may not be able to communicate their needs effectively, and physiological responses are attenuated by illness and treatments, so consider use of short acting agents and assess response to incremental doses. Reassuringly, patients who become delirium free after stopping sedation have the same prognosis as patients without delirium. We should also pay attention to normalising physiology where possible, especially aiming for normal oxygen and carbon dioxide levels and a well-hydrated status.

NON-PHARMACOLOGICAL MANAGEMENT

Environmental factors can be controlled to reduce the risk of delirium. ICUs are noisy, with ventilators, filters and alarms all contributing to background and peak noise levels. However, this should be kept to a minimum when possible and especially overnight by setting alarm levels appropriately, responding to them promptly and avoiding unnecessary conversation near bed spaces.

A normal sleep-wake cycle should be promoted by altering lighting overnight, and attempting to reduce noise and activity overnight, for example by grouping activities around the bedspace to minimise disturbances, and offering patients earplugs and masks. During the day, the patient should be frequently re-orientated using repetitive, simple explanations, and engage with physiotherapy and the nursing staff to undertake normal daytime behaviour.

Maximise communication with the patient by ensuring hearing aids have batteries and are turned on, glasses are clean and appropriate, and providing means of non-verbal communication for patients with tracheostomies. Consider providing a clock or calendar within easy view of the bedspace, and allowing a patient's family to bring photographs and other memorabilia to the bedspace to allow the patient to re-orientate themselves.

If a patient does become delirious, management should be holistic, and focused primarily on explaining what is happening to both the patient and their relatives. Many patients are concerned they are 'going mad' and need reassurance that delirium is a commonly experienced aspect of critical illness, rather than a permanent psychiatric disease from which they will never recover. Relatives too often need reassurance that delirium is part of critical illness, and that they can play a role in resolution through orientation, relieving anxiety, and sleep promotion. Also consider and correct other causes for agitation such as pain, hypoxia and hypoglycaemia.

PHARMACOLOGICAL MANAGEMENT

Antipsychotic therapy is the mainstay of medical management, but needs to be used in concert with the above personal and environmental measures to be successful. Haloperidol is the recommended first-line agent, but should be used in caution for patients with prolonged QT interval, and avoided in patients with Parkinson's due to their susceptibility to extra-pyramidal side effects (which can affect any patient and are treated with procyclidine).

Although patients may appear to respond to a bolus dose, their delirium is unlikely to resolve immediately, so regular therapy with PRN 'breakthrough' cover is often appropriate. Rarely an infusion can be considered for severe delirium. Atypical antipsychotics such as quetiapine, risperidone and olanzapine are alternatives, and may have a preferable side effect profile, especially in those who have experienced or are prone to the side effects of haloperidol.

Very occasionally, patients may need rapid sedation to prevent them from becoming a risk to themselves or others; however, routine sedation is counterproductive in avoiding delirium in the longer term.

Patients who are severely agitated and becoming a risk of harm to themselves or others may require restraints, either in the form of 'mitts' or 'boxing gloves', or to prevent them from lashing out with limbs. This should be performed in the least restrictive manner, with the patient's capacity regularly assessed and consideration as to the use of a Deprivation of Liberty Safeguards (DoLS) form.

Often patients will initially respond well to a bolus medication but then appear to relapse; remember that delirium is by nature a fluctuating condition, so brief periods of normality may be falsely reassuring. Continue therapy until two consecutive, twelve-hourly negative assessments are achieved and an episode of delirium can be said to have 'resolved'.

CASE RESOLUTION

You ensure that Mr Smith has no other biological cause for agitation and that his pain is well controlled. His RASS is +1 and he is CAM-ICU positive when you screen him, so you make the diagnosis of hyperactive critical care delirium. You encourage the nursing staff to regularly orientate Mr Smith and promote a healthy sleep-wake cycle, and after a PRN haloperidol dose, he seems a lot more settled, so you prescribe him regular haloperidol and ask for his CAM-ICU score to be checked in twelve hours time. Two days later, his delirium has resolved and he is discharged to the ward.

KEY LEARNING POINTS

- Delirium is common sequelae to critical illness and a cause of increased morbidity and mortality, yet is easily reversible as long as you look for it!
- Mainstay of management is holistic – reassure your patients that they are experiencing a transient part of critical illness, rather than a permanent psychiatric state.
- When prescribing sedatives, ask yourself: are you giving this for the patient's benefit, or to make your life easier?

FURTHER READING

Girard, Timothy D., Pratik P. Pandharipande, and E. Wesley Ely. "Delirium in the Intensive Care Unit." *Critical Care* 12, suppl. 3 (May 2008): S3.

Inouye, Sharon K., Christopher H. van Dyck, Cathy A. Alessi, Sharyl Balkin, Alan P. Siegal, and Ralph I. Horwitz. "Clarifying Confusion: The Confusion Assessment Method. A New Method for Detection of Delirium." *Annals of Internal Medicine* 113, no. 12 (December 1990): 941–948.

National Institute for Health and Care Excellence. "Delirium: Diagnosis, Prevention and Management." Clinical guideline CG103, National Institute for Health and Care Excellence, Manchester, UK, July 2010 (updated January 2015).

VUMC Center for Health Services Research, Vanderbilt University. "ICU Delirium and Cognitive Impairment Study Group." www.icudelirium .org (accessed 10 November 2017).

33

Status epilepticus

BRYONY PATRICK AND ANDREW GOSLING

'Please can you come to see this patient? She arrived in the Emergency Department ten minutes ago having a seizure and there's been no improvement.'

Recognition and management of seizures is an important topic in intensive care medicine, as we often care for patient groups at high risk for convulsions. This may include patients with pre-existing epilepsy and intra-cranial pathologies such as tumours, or less obvious factors such as alcohol withdrawal. Status epilepticus is a medical emergency due to the risk of permanent brain damage and should be approached using the 'ABCDE' method to ensure patient safety. Seizures can be frightening to witness, especially for family members, so a calm logical approach to diagnosis and treatment is important.

DEFINITION

Five minutes or more of convulsions OR two or more convulsions in a five-minute period without return to preconvulsion neurological baseline.

This has been updated from the traditional definition of 30 minutes of seizure activity as

- Significant brain injury can happen within half an hour.
- Most seizures that do not progress to status will last less than five minutes.
- Early drug treatment is most effective at terminating seizure activity.

Note that a patient who has not 'woken up' following a single seizure may be in status; further investigations may be needed to diagnose this.

Non-convulsive status epilepticus (seizure activity seen on EEG only) is also relevant to the ICU population. It is typically seen in patients with severely impaired mental status, for example following a traumatic brain injury and can be difficult to diagnose due to the lack of clinical signs. It carries a high mortality rate (61%).

CAUSES

Seizures account for about a third of neurological presentations and 1% of Emergency Department attendances, and there is significant overall morbidity and mortality associated with status epilepticus. Around 20% of patients do not survive to leave the hospital and around 15% are left with severe neurological or cognitive problems.

There are multiple causes for seizures, both acute and chronic.

ACUTE

- Metabolic disturbance – electrolyte abnormalities, hypoglycaemia, renal failure
- Infection – sepsis, CNS infection, e.g. meningitis, encephalitis or abscess

- Vascular – cerebrovascular accident (ischaemic or haemorrhagic), subarachnoid haemorrhage, venous sinus thrombosis, severe hypertension
- Head injury
- Toxins – drug induced, alcohol/benzodiazepine/opioid withdrawal
- Hypoxia – cardiac arrest
- Polypharmacy – e.g. drug interaction with ongoing anti-epileptic medication
- Other – autoimmune encephalitis, paraneoplastic syndromes

CHRONIC

- Structural – central nervous system (CNS) tumours
- Epilepsy – including noncompliance with medication
- Pseudoseizures (dissociative seizures)
  - Psychologically mediated
    - Suggestive signs: gradual onset, fluctuating motor activity with violent limb movements, pelvic thrusting movements and lateral head movements, rapid recovery, resistance to eye opening, normal pupils and plantar reflexes

The history (often limited to collateral history from witnesses) is therefore vital.

MANAGEMENT

AIRWAY AND BREATHING

This may be threatened by reduced conscious level and secretions or bleeding from oral trauma, e.g. tongue biting. The airway may well be difficult to manage during generalised seizure activity so consider basic measures such as applying facemask oxygen and oral suctioning of secretions as able. Position the patient on their side if/when possible to reduce the risk of aspiration and consider inserting a nasopharyngeal airway (NPA) to relieve signs of airway obstruction. The arterial blood gas (ABG) findings usually show a mixed respiratory and metabolic acidosis due to poor ventilation during a seizure and high metabolic demand of skeletal muscles. Patients may need intubation and ventilation to protect the airway and control oxygenation.

CIRCULATION

Flushing, hypertension and tachycardia are often seen during early seizure activity due to sympathetic stimulation, followed by hypotension. Give fluids as needed and review the need for vasoactive drugs to maintain normal blood pressure and ensure brain perfusion. Regarding intervention, it is important to swiftly obtain good IV access and send baseline bloods including arterial or venous blood gas early to help identify the underlying cause. Note the white cell count is often raised following seizure activity so it should not be viewed in isolation to diagnose an infective cause.

DISABILITY

Pupils are typically dilated and reactive in seizures; unequal and/or unreactive pupils may suggest an intracranial pathology. Observe tonic–clonic movements, which may become less pronounced as the seizure continues due to muscle fatigue. It is crucial to check the blood glucose level and give dextrose if low (<3 mmol/L), but remember the blood glucose can initially be high and then drop so it will need repeating. A CT head will often be performed to look for an intracranial cause unless the precipitating cause is very obvious and there is a low risk of secondary trauma. Treatment measures focus on minimising potential further neuronal damage by reducing the intracranial pressure (ICP). This can be done by sitting the patient slightly head up if safe to do so and ensuring that clothing and equipment around the neck is not too tight. Also, consider giving thiamine (250 mg as Pabrinex) if there is a suspicion of alcohol abuse or poor nutrition.

EXAMINATION

As part of our standard observations, we should check the patient's temperature (commonly slightly raised due to increased metabolic rate). You will need to perform a thorough head to toe examination looking for indications to the underlying cause and any associated injuries.

DRUG TREATMENT

This depends on the setting and clinical picture. Pre-hospital teams or sometimes family members are often the first to deliver an anticonvulsant; it is important to know what and how much of it has been given. *The critical factor in predicting ease of controlling seizure activity is time to administering anticonvulsants.* In a hospital setting, the following regime is generally used:

- Lorazepam (0.1 mg/kg) up to 4 mg IV over about 2 minutes can be repeated after 10 minutes.
    - Alternatively, diazepam 5 mg IV/10–20 mg PR ('diazemuls')
    - Or midazolam 10 mg buccal
- Ensure any regular anti-epileptic medication is given.
- Phenytoin 'loading dose' 15–18 mg/kg at a rate of 50 mg/min.
    - Alternatively, fosphenytoin IV (prodrug with less hypotensive effects, 1.5 mg = 1 mg phenytoin) 15–20 mg phenytoin equivalents (PE) at 50–100 mg PE/min.
    - Or phenobarbital IV 10–15 mg/kg at 100 mg/min.
    - Or valproic acid IV 40 mg/kg over 10 min.
    - Phenytoin and phenobarbital can be continued at maintenance doses guided by the serum levels.
- General anaesthetic with thiopentone or propofol bolus and continued as an infusion.
    - Consider midazolam infusion.
    - Sedation continued for 12–24 hours after end of seizure activity then slowly weaned down.
    - Avoid use of long acting neuromuscular blockers in order to observe for evidence of further seizures.

FURTHER INVESTIGATIONS

These aim to identify the underlying cause and any complications and may include the following:

- Electrocardiography (ECG)
- Chest X-ray (CXR) – for infection, neurogenic pulmonary oedema and signs of aspiration
- Toxicology screen (urine)
- Electroencephalography (EEG) monitoring
- CT/MRI brain – then relevant discussion with neurology or neurosurgical teams if required
- Lumbar puncture – consider starting prophylactic broad spectrum antibiotics and antivirals
- Blood cultures

CLINICAL CASE

You attend the emergency department to find a 21-year-old woman having a tonic-clonic seizure. She is accompanied by her mother who reports she is known to be epileptic but has missed her medication for the last two days as she has been vomiting. The patient had a seizure earlier in the day for which she delivered her 'rescue' diazemul and phoned the ambulance. The seizure seemed to stop but has started again on arrival in Emergency and she has received a further 4 mg of IV lorazepam. They have taken a set of baseline bloods but the results are not available as of yet.

On assessing the patient you find:

HR 138 sinus tachycardia
BP 150/98
Saturation 93% on 15 L non-rebreathe mask
Tonic–clonic movements with bilaterally dilated pupils that respond to light
Noisy sounding breathing with lots of oral secretions

Actions:

Call for help early on!
A – turn onto side if possible, insert NPA and continue with 15 L non-rebreathe mask
B – assess respiratory pattern and depth, listen to the chest, ABG – shows pH 7.30, PO_2 8, $PaCO_2$ 7, Lactate 4
C – Repeat observations; stable
D – BM = 13 mmol/L

You decide to give a second dose of lorazepam intravenously but there is no improvement over the next five minutes. You are concerned that her breathing pattern seems to be worsening and her saturations are now 90%. The emergency doctor has checked the dose of phenytoin and prescribed the infusion appropriately. Whilst the nurse is drawing it up, you see vomit draining onto the pillow from the patient's mouth and you are unable to pass the suction into her mouth as her jaw is clenched. You call for help from the anaesthetic team on call, recognising that the patient's airway is compromised and she now requires intubation.

She is intubated and started on a propofol infusion for maintenance of anaesthesia. You arrange for transfer to ICU for observation after discussing with the consultant on call, deciding that she does not need a CT head as the cause is evident and there are no signs of trauma on examination.

She is admitted to the ICU where EEG monitoring is sited. Her admission bloods show electrolyte derangement in keeping with a history of vomiting, which are replaced to normal levels. The white cell count (WCC) is raised as expected but she continues to spike fevers. She is started on antibiotics for aspiration pneumonia as the chest X-ray shows infiltrates at the right base. On discussion with the neurology team, her regular dose of sodium valproate is restarted and the sedation level is weaned down the following day before being extubated.

KEY LEARNING POINTS

- The ABCDE assessment should be used when approaching a patient with seizures.
- Take a good history from witnesses, especially the pre-hospital team who you will not be able to question at a later point.
- Prompt treatment with anticonvulsant medication is imperative.
- It is important to thoroughly assess potential trigger factors; these may also need treating for resolution of status epilepticus to occur.

FURTHER READING

Brophy, Gretchen M., Rodney Bell, Jan Claassen, Brian Alldredge, Thomas P. Bleck, Tracy Glauser, Suzette M. LaRoche, James J. Riviello Jr., Lori Shutter, Michael R. Sperling, David M. Treiman, and Paul M. Vespa, for the Neurocritical Care Society Status Epilepticus Guideline Writing Committee. "Guidelines for the Evaluation and Management of Status Epilepticus." *Neurocritical Care* 17 (April 2012): 3–23. www.mc.vanderbilt .edu/documents/NeuroICU/files/Status.pdf (accessed 20 June 2017).

Cadogan, Mike, and Chris Nickson. 2016. "Status Epilepticus." *Life in the Fast Lane.* https://lifeinthefastlane.com/ccc/status-epilepticus/ (accessed 24 June 2017).

National Institute for Health and Care Excellence. "Treating Prolonged or Repeated Seizures and Convulsive Status Epilepticus - NICE Pathways." https://pathways.nice.org.uk/pathways/epilepsy/treating-prolonged

-or-repeated-seizures-and-convulsive-status-epilepticus (accessed 24 June 2017).

Neurocritical Care Society. "Status Epilepticus." *ENLS: Emergency Neurological Life Support.* http://enlsprotocols.org:8080/protocols/enls-body .html?id=15## (accessed 24 June 2017).

34

The critically ill or injured child in a non-paediatric hospital

ELDILLA RIZAL AND NITIN ARORA

You receive a 'paediatric alert' call in the Resuscitation Bay in the Emergency Department (ED). When you arrive, you meet Angel Smith: a 3-month-old brought in by ambulance with respiratory distress, poor feeding and lethargy. She had been unwell for 48 hours with coryzal symptoms but had been unable to feed and had not passed any urine for 24 hours. On examination, she is mottled, and in significant respiratory distress and has a prolonged apnoea despite being stimulated. The paediatric doctor asks you for help. What do you do?

As an intensive care doctor in a hospital without tertiary paediatric support, this is not an uncommon situation especially in the winter months. It can be very daunting to be called to a paediatric emergency as this is out of your comfort zone and is in a different department to your own. Furthermore, the situation is often stressful for even the most experienced ED staff.

However, by the end of reading this chapter, you may be equipped with a systematic approach to managing a critically ill or injured child whilst awaiting a tertiary retrieval team. An important thing to remember is that you are never alone and you should use the resources available to you – the local paediatric team, your consultant, operating department practitioner (ODP) and paediatric nursing staff. Being sensitive and professional is key to maintaining trust in one's local hospital.

WHAT DO CRITICALLY ILL CHILDREN PRESENT TO DISTRICT GENERAL HOSPITALS WITH?

There are 34 Paediatric Intensive Care Units (PICUs) in the UK reflecting centralisation of specialist care. In 2014, 6000 children required transferring to a hospital with a PICU and 77% of them were transferred by a specialist paediatric intensive care and retrieval team (PICANET 2015 report).

The majority of children requiring PICU are under one year of age with mainly respiratory ailments including bronchiolitis and pneumonia.

Potential diagnoses of critically ill children can include the following:

RESPIRATORY CONDITIONS

- Bronchiolitis
- Epiglottitis (Call ENT!)
- Near drowning

CARDIAC CONDITIONS

- Myocarditis

SEPSIS

- Meningococcal septicaemia

NEUROLOGICAL CONDITIONS

- Status epilepticus
- Head injury

NON-ACCIDENTAL INJURY (NAI)

- Physical abuse and neglect

RECOGNITION OF THE CRITICALLY ILL CHILD

Paediatric physiological parameters vary with age. See table below.

Other signs of an unwell child include lethargy, mottling, cool peripheries, reduced urine output and altered consciousness. (Note a febrile child can display these signs but have a remarkable response to antipyretics.)

	Respiratory Rate	Heart Rate	Systolic BP (50th Centile)
Infants 0–11 m	30–60	90–160	60–90
Preschool 1–4 y	20–40	90–140	80–100
School 5–13 y	20–30	70–120	90–110
Teenage 13–18 y	10–20	60–100	90–140

INVESTIGATIONS

BLOODS

- Full blood count
- Urea and electrolytes
- Liver function tests
- Blood gas – capillary, venous or arterial
- Blood culture
- Meningococcal PCR (if appropriate)

URINE

- Microscopy and culture
- Toxicology (if NAI suspected)

OTHER INVESTIGATIONS

Lumbar puncture may be indicated if meningitis is suspected and the patient is not coagulopathic. Take three samples in sterile universal containers and send for microscopy and culture, protein, viral PCR and another sample in a grey-top bottle for glucose and lactate.

Chest X-ray will be indicated to check ET position and for pneumonia. (NB: Broken ribs can sometimes be missed in NAI when looking for other pathology.)

WHAT DO YOU DO IN THIS EMERGENCY SITUATION? (MANAGEMENT OF CRITICALLY ILL CHILD)

Remember your ABCs

1. Ensure patent airway. Give 100% oxygen.
2. Bag, valve and mask at 30 breaths per minute to achieve effective ventilation. Watch for chest rise and improvement in oxygen saturations.

3. Get the ODP/nurse to prepare intubation drugs and equipment (including emergency drugs). Ensure the paediatric team is liaising (or has liaised) with the regional paediatric retrieval service as you are about to intubate this child and they will need an appropriate definitive place of care – a PICU! Call your consultant if you haven't already done so.
4. Obtain IV access. If struggling (>2 attempts), insert an IO needle. Treat for sepsis with a broad-spectrum antibiotic like cefotaxime. This is time critical and can be lifesaving.
5. Maintain sedation and anaesthesia until retrieval team arrives.
6. Document findings and actions clearly.
7. Ensure there is ongoing dialogue with the retrieval/accepting team.

The likely diagnosis is bronchiolitis. The child is likely to require intubation, ventilation and transfer to PICU. Apnoeas can also be a feature of sepsis and therefore it is best to administer antibiotics. The history of poor feeding and mottling suggests impending circulatory decompensation and thus will need IV fluids, and possibly inotropic support.

The goal of your management is to stabilise the child by securing the airway, ventilating effectively and ensuring a well-filled circulation, in preparation for transfer to PICU.

AIRWAY CONSIDERATIONS

The main indications for intubation include apnoea, decreased respiratory drive, ineffective respiration, lung failure, and airways obstruction (epiglottitis), to reduce the work of breathing in a critically ill child with septic shock or cardiac failure.

Uncuffed endotracheal tubes should be used in infants, while cuffed tubes should be used in older children.

Paediatric airways are positionally anterior compared with the adult. Optimise positioning with a 'sniffing the morning air' approach. Infants have relatively larger occiputs and a shoulder roll is often helpful.

Their mucosa and skin are also more susceptible to trauma, so caution should be exercised.

Below is a rough guide of ET tube sizes and positions:

	Size of ETT (mm)	Length at lips (cm)	Length at nostril (cm)
Preterm	2.5–3	6–8	Not recommended
Neonate – 6 m	3.5–4	9–11	11–13
6–12 m	4–4.5	10–12	12–15
1–2 y	4.5–5	11–13	14–16
>2 y	Age (years)/4 + 4	Age (years)/2 + 12	Age (years)/2 + 15

Fixation of the tube is crucial in children. Small movements of the head and neck in an infant can mean inadvertent extubation or intubation of the right main bronchus! The ODP will be familiar with the locally preferred technique.

SEDATIVE AND MUSCLE RELAXATION DRUGS AND DOSES

Sedative Drugs	Induction Dose	Dose per 50 mL of 0.9% NaCl/ D5/D10	Suggested Dose and Rate of Infusion
Ketamine	1–2 mg/kg		
Fentanyl	1–5 mcg/kg		
Thiopentone	2–4 mg/kg		
Propofol	1–5 mg//kg		
Morphine		3 mg/kg	10–40 mcg/kg/hr 1–2 mL/hr
Midazolam		3 mg/kg	0.5–1 mcg/kg/min

VENTILATION

Transport ventilators are often basic pneumatic ventilators. Familiarise yourself with the kit before an emergency situation arises.

Differences in paediatric lung physiology are a result of narrower airways, increased airway resistance, compliant chest walls, horizontal ribs and lower functional residual capacity. Children have fewer functional alveoli, and have a tendency to de-recruit and decompensate quickly.

Neuro-Muscular Blocking Drugs	Intubation Dose	Dose per 50 mL	Suggested Dose and Rate of Infusion
Rocuronium	0.6–1 mg/kg	Neat solution (100 mg/10 mL)	0.5–1 mg/kg/hr
Atracurium	0.3–0.6 mg/kg		0.3–1.7 mg/kg/hr
Suxamethonium	Weight <10 kg 2 mg/kg Weight > = 10 kg 1 mg/kg		
Vecuronium	0.1 mg/kg	6 mg/kg	1–4 mcg/kg/min

Mechanical ventilation should be considered if there are clinical features of respiratory distress such as grunting, tachypnoea, accessory muscle use, tachycardia or bradycardia, impaired consciousness, cyanosis or exhaustion. Objective measures can also be used and include FiO_2 >0.6, respiratory acidosis, PaO_2/FiO_2 <20 and oxygenation index >13.

Sample initial ventilator settings are as follows:

	Preterm	Neonate	1–5 y	5–12 y	>12 y
PIP (cmH$_2$O)	20	15	n/a	n/a	n/a
PEEP (cmH$_2$O)	5	4–10	4–10	4–15	4–15
V$_T$ (mL/kg)	4–6	5–10	5–10	5–10	5–10
Rate	40–60	25–40	20–25	15–20	12–15
I:E	1:1	1:2	1:2	1:2	1:2
Ti (secs)	0.4–0.5	0.65–0.8	0.8–1	1–1.2	1.5

SUPPORTING THE CIRCULATION

In an acutely unwell child, it is acceptable to give fluid boluses in the remit of 20 mL/kg of crystalloid or colloid. Once you have given 40 mL/kg, expect that respiratory distress will ensue and you will need to be prepared to secure a definitive airway. In trauma, use 10 mL/kg aliquots.

If several fluid boluses are required to maintain adequate circulation, and the retrieval team is still en route, it can be helpful to consider peripheral strength adrenaline to run in the background during intubation. The table below is a guide on how these drugs can be prescribed and made up peripherally.

Peripheral Inotropes	Dose per 50 mL	Suggested Dose and Rate of Infusion
Adrenaline	0.3 mg/kg but up to maximum of 1 mg	0.01–1 mcg/kg/min
Noradrenaline	0.3 mg/kg up to maximum of 1 mg	0.01–1 mcg/kg/min
Dopamine	80 mg	5–20 mcg/kg/min
Dobutamine	80 mg	5–20 mcg/kg/min

HUMAN FACTORS

Managing critically ill children involves a wide variety of expertise and necessitates effective communication. It is vital to include parents in the picture, and it can be pertinent to have a member of staff supporting them.

KEY LEARNING POINTS

- Children do present critically ill in district general hospitals and it is not unusual for ICU doctors to be asked for assistance. It is important to keep up your skills in managing children from the beginning.
- Remember to use the ABC approach using the relevant considerations as above.
- Use your local resources wisely and always involve consultant support. Always look up drug doses, and use a calculator!
- Remember that NAI can present in an abundance of ways and to be mindful of this; also, make the appropriate referral to the designated team at your hospital.

FURTHER READING

Barry, Peter, Kevin Morris, and Tariq Ali (Eds.). *Paediatric Intensive Care (Oxford Specialist Handbooks in Paediatrics).* Oxford: Oxford University Press; 2010.

Department of Health (UK). *The Acutely or Critically Sick or Injured Child in the District General Hospital.* Closed consultation. http://webarchive .nationalarchives.gov.uk/+/www.dh.gov.uk/en/Consultations /Closedconsultations/DH_4124412 (accessed 13 February 2017).

Paediatric Intensive Care Audit Network (Universities of Leeds and Leicester). "Paediatric Intensive Care Audit Network (PICANet) - Home." www.picanet.org.uk (accessed 13 February 2017).

35

Management of hyperglycaemic emergencies

BEN WOOLDRIDGE AND PAUL JOHNSTON

Mr Evans, a type-1 diabetic, is admitted to the Emergency Department (ED) drowsy and breathless, complaining of extreme thirst. His blood ketones are high and an arterial blood gas reveals a severe metabolic acidosis. The ED doctors have made a diagnosis of diabetic ketoacidosis (DKA) and have requested you to review the patient as they would like advice on the management of his condition.

WHAT IS DIABETIC KETOACIDOSIS?

DKA is an abnormal metabolic state caused by a deficiency in insulin leading to a triad of clinical features:

- Hyperglycaemia
- Ketonaemia
- Acidosis

In the absence of insulin, the body responds by the production of growth hormone, cortisol and glucagon. These hormones initiate the following metabolic processes:

- Glycogenolysis – the break down of body glycogen stores to glucose
- Gluconeogenesis – production of glucose from non-carbohydrate precursors
- Lipolysis – breakdown of triglycerides to free fatty acids and glycerol

The increase in glucose production leads to severe hyperglycaemia and the breakdown of fatty acids as an alternative form of energy produces ketone bodies causing a metabolic acidosis.

EPIDEMIOLOGY

DKA is a common condition seen throughout all NHS hospitals in the United Kingdom, not infrequently requiring admission to intensive care.

In 2014, 14,375 patients were admitted to hospital in the United Kingdom with DKA and 13% required intensive care support. Our increased understanding of the pathophysiology of DKA has led to better treatment and reduced mortality over the last 20 years.

WHAT CAUSES DKA?

- Infection/sepsis – pneumonia, urinary tract infection, intra-abdominal sepsis
- Inappropriate insulin treatment
- Excessive alcohol consumption
- New diagnosis of diabetes mellitus

WHAT ARE THE CLINICAL FEATURES?

DKA predominantly affects patients who suffer from type-1 diabetes. However, patients with type-2 diabetes who are prone to the development of ketosis can also develop the condition.

Symptoms and signs include

- Polyuria
- Polydipsia
- Tiredness/lethargy
- Nausea and vomiting
- Abdominal pain
- Kussmaul breathing
- Reduced consciousness

HOW CAN A DIAGNOSIS OF DKA BE CONFIRMED IN MR EVANS?

Investigations should aim to confirm the diagnosis of DKA and then establish the underlying cause.

The following features must be present to confirm DKA:

1. Ketonaemia ≥ 3 mmol/L or significant ketonuria (> 2+ on urine sticks)
2. Blood glucose > 11 mmol/L or known diabetes mellitus
3. Bicarbonate < 15 mmol/L, venous pH < 7.3, or both

A detailed clinical history and performing a full systems examination is essential in finding the underlying cause of DKA. Baseline investigations should be performed and should include

- Full blood count/CRP
- Urea and electrolytes
- Liver function tests
- Amylase
- Blood cultures
- ECG
- Pregnancy test

HOW SHOULD MR EVANS BE MANAGED?

Remember ABCDE: ensure the airway is protected, give oxygen and establish intravenous access. Treatment should then be directed to the following key areas.

FLUID RESUSCITATION

Administration of appropriate fluid to a patient suffering with DKA is the most important therapeutic intervention. Either 0.9% saline or balanced electrolyte solution can be used with appropriate potassium replacement as necessary. Concern has been raised regarding the use of 0.9% saline due to its chloride content and its potential to cause a hyperchloraemic acidosis. However, the National Patient Safety Agency has recognised that 0.9% saline is a fluid that is familiar to physicians and readily available on all wards. It is available in bags containing a predetermined concentration of potassium unlike a balanced electrolyte solution that would require potassium to be added to the bag separately, increasing the risk of drug errors. In view of this, it is recommended that 0.9% saline is the fluid of choice for use on medical wards when treating DKA. In a critical care environment, however, a balanced electrolyte solution is often the preferred fluid of choice and administration of potassium either peripherally or centrally is commonplace. It is therefore entirely appropriate to use a balanced electrolyte solution in this clinical setting.

HYPERGLYCAEMIA

A fixed rate insulin infusion calculated according to patient weight (0.1 unit/kg/hr) should be administered to treat hyperglycaemia. Fifty units of Actrapid diluted in 50 mL of 0.9% saline to give a final concentration of 1 unit mL should be prepared. The therapeutic targets used in order to monitor response to treatment are as follows:

- Reduction in blood ketone concentration by >0.5 mmol/L/h
- Increase in venous bicarbonate by 3 mmol/L/h
- Reduction in capillary blood glucose by 3 mmol/L/h

Failure of these targets to be achieved raises suspicion that insufficient insulin is being administered. There are a number of factors that should be considered:

- An appropriate concentration of insulin is being delivered to the patient.
- Insulin is being transfused and the syringe driver is working correctly.
- The cannula being used to deliver the infusion is working.

If an insufficient concentration of insulin is being administered to the patient, the infusion rate can be increased by 1 unit per hour. A maximum rate of 15 units per hour of Actrapid should not be exceeded.

Capillary blood glucose levels can be checked hourly. If the glucose level falls below 14 mmol/L, supplementary 10% glucose is recommended at a rate of 125 mL/h. Care must be taken not to overload the patient with fluid.

ADMINISTRATION OF ELECTROLYTES

Serum potassium levels in the body will fall as the insulin infusion is commenced. During the initial resuscitation period, potassium should not be added to the fluid if the serum level is above 5.5 mmol/L. If the serum potassium levels are below 5.5 mmol/L and the patient is passing urine, then it should be replaced by giving 0.9% sodium chloride containing 40 mmol of potassium. In cases of severe hypokalaemia, critical care input is required to consider central venous potassium replacement.

HOW SHOULD MR EVANS' FLUID REGIMEN BE PRESCRIBED?

A typical fluid regimen can be seen in the table below for a 70-kg individual with DKA. However, every patient is different and underlying comorbidities must be taken into consideration and the fluid prescription adjusted accordingly to avoid fluid overload.

Fluid	Volume
0.9% Sodium Chloride	1000 mL over 1 hour
0.9% Sodium Chloride + Potassium Chloride	1000 mL over 2 hours
0.9% Sodium Chloride + Potassium Chloride	1000 mL over 2 hours
0.9% Sodium Chloride + Potassium Chloride	1000 mL over 4 hours
0.9% Sodium Chloride + Potassium Chloride	1000 mL over 4 hours
0.9% Sodium Chloride + Potassium Chloride	1000 mL over 6 hours

OTHER CONSIDERATIONS

- *Urethral catheterisation* – in patients who are oliguric or have evidence of acute kidney injury
- *Venous thromboembolism prophylaxis*
- *Antibiotics* – only indicated in patients with evidence of infection

DOES MR EVANS REQUIRE ADMISSION TO CRITICAL CARE?

Critical care involvement is recommended when any of the following features are present indicating severe DKA:

- GCS < 12
- Severe acidosis (pH < 7.1)
- Bicarbonate levels < 5 mmol/L
- Hypotension (systolic < 90 mmHg)
- Hypokalaemia < 3.5 mmol/L

COMPLICATIONS OF DKA

CEREBRAL OEDEMA

Occurs more commonly in children and young adults (18–25 years of age), the exact underlying cause of which is unclear. In the event of a patient showing symptoms and signs of raised intracranial pressure reduce the rate of intravenous fluid resuscitation, acquire expert help and consider the use of hypertonic saline and mannitol. A CT head is mandatory to exclude alternative pathology.

PULMONARY OEDEMA

A rare complication usually associated with poor underlying cardiac function. Critical care input may be required where large volume fluid resuscitation may prove problematic to allow central venous monitoring and targeted fluid replacement.

HYPOGLYCAEMIA

Occurs following commencement of the fixed rate insulin infusion that can lead to a number of complications including cerebral impairment, arrhythmias and rebound ketosis.

IMPORTANT POINTS FOR CONSIDERATION

1. Monitoring response to treatment can be achieved by taking venous blood gases.
2. Measurement of blood ketone levels during treatment is important, as it is the best investigation to monitor response to treatment.
3. Long acting insulin should be continued in patients already on treatment. Short acting insulin analogues should be stopped.
4. Intravenous bicarbonate is not indicated as it causes a rise in carbon dioxide partial pressure within cerebrospinal fluid (CSF) causing a CSF acidosis.

FOLLOWING TREATMENT

Resolution of DKA is defined as a pH > 7.3 and blood ketones < 3 mmol/L. At this point, the insulin infusion can be stopped and conversion back to subcutaneous insulin can take place. Consultation with the diabetes specialist team and patient education should take place to prevent further episodes in the future.

HOW IS DKA DIFFERENT FROM HYPEROSMOLAR HYPERGLYCAEMIC STATE (HHS)?

HHS is characterised by evidence of hypovolaemia, hyperglycaemia (> 30 mmol/L) without ketonaemia or acidosis and a plasma osmolality of > 320 mOsm/kg. It has a higher mortality that DKA and its treatment is different. HHS typically develops over a longer period and therefore the metabolic disturbances are greater and complications such as thromboembolic disease, cerebral oedema and seizures are greater. Treatment involves restoration of circulating volume, correction of hyperglycaemia and thromboprophylaxis.

KEY LEARNING POINTS

- DKA is a common presenting condition in hospitals and if not treated appropriately mortality is high.
- Diagnosis is based on history, examination and basic investigations.
- Appropriate fluid resuscitation is the most important therapeutic intervention.
- Blood ketones should be used to monitor response to treatment, **NOT** resolution of hyperglycaemia.
- All patients should be reviewed by the diabetic specialist team prior to discharge.

FURTHER READING

Hallett, Abbie, and Nicholas Levy. "Developments in the Management of Diabetic Ketoacidosis in Adults: Implications for Anaethetists." *BJA Education* 16, no. 1 (January 2016): 8–14.

Joint British Diabetes Societies Inpatient Care Group, *The Management of Diabetic Ketoacidosis in Adults*, March 2010, www.bsped.org.uk /clinical/docs/dkamanagementofdkainadultsmarch20101.pdf (accessed 13 February 2017).

Joint British Diabetes Societies Inpatient Care Group, *The Management of the Hyperosmolar Hyperglycaemic State (HHS) in Adults with Diabetes*, August 2012, www.diabetologists-abcd.org.uk/JBDS/JBDS_IP_HHS _Adults.pdf (accessed 13 February 2017).

Rudd, Bryony, Krishna Patel, Nicholas Levy, and Ketan Dhatariya. "A Survey of the Implementation of NHS Diabetes Guidelines for Management of Diabetic Ketoacidosis in the Intensive Care Units of the East of England." *Journal of the Intensive Care Society* 14, no. 1 (January 2013): 60–64.

36

Poisoning

NAGENDRA PINNAMPENI AND ARUMUGAM JAGADEESWARAN

Acute poisoning is one of the commonest medical emergencies. There are specific antidotes available for some poisons and drugs, but the majority of the management is supportive and recovery will follow. TOXBASE (www.toxbase.org) is the best resource for managing acute poisoning; check with your Emergency Department (ED) about login details for your hospital. Unfortunately, there is no universally accepted algorithm to aid in evaluation. Contact your local poison centre (Poisons Information Service, UK 0844 892 0111) when in doubt.

GENERAL MEASURES

1. The most important management available at present is supportive care.
2. Always remember your **ABCDE**.

3. **Airway & Breathing** – Support the airway if the patients are drowsy and intubate the comatose and seizing patients. Tracheal intubation and airway protection is almost always necessary when a patient tolerates insertion of an oropharyngeal airway, so *call for help.*

4. **Circulation** – Establish venous access, and treat hypotension initially with volume expansion. Basic observations, including blood pressure, pulse rate, peripheral perfusion and urine output should be recorded.

5. **Disability** – Monitor trend of the patient's Glasgow Coma Scale (GCS) and act based on it. If GCS < 8, ask for help to obtain a definitive airway for two reasons:
   a. To prevent aspiration
   b. To prevent respiratory acidosis, as it increases the risk of arrhythmias

6. **Exposure & Environment** – Observe your safety if you do not know about the overdose. Expose the patient to rule out other injuries and prevent hypothermia.

7. **Investigations** – Important initial investigations include:
   a. Basic biochemistry – many drugs depend on renal elimination. Renal insufficiency may alter the management. Glucose and liver function tests need to be reviewed.
   b. Urinalysis – urine toxicology as appropriate, with a sample kept for later analysis if required.
   c. ABG analysis – metabolic/respiratory acidosis is most common. Management of those are important.
   d. Chest X-ray – to rule out inhalation of gastric contents.
   e. Drug levels – very helpful in specific poisons, e.g. paracetamol, salicylates, iron, digoxin and lithium.

8. **Gut Decontamination** – Not valid for most of the time. Useful if performed within **one hour** of drug ingestion. If performed later, the amount of poison removed is insignificant, and lavage may only propel unabsorbed poison into small intestine. Prior intubation is essential when airway is in doubt.
   a. Tepid tap water through large-bore tube (36–40 Fr).
   b. Activated charcoal – highly effective in adsorbing many toxins due to its large surface area and porous structure. Works effectively if given within one hour of ingestion.

9. **Enhancing Drug Elimination** – Useful in limited number of poisonings.
   a. Urinary alkalinisation, e.g. salicylates
   b. Extracorporeal techniques, e.g. haemodialysis, haemoperfusion – specifically used for poisoning from ethylene glycol, lithium, methanol, phenobarbital, salicylates and sodium valproate
10. Continue supportive care with attention paid to fluid balance, correction of electrolytes, initiation of nutritional support and prompt treatment of nosocomial infection.
11. Psychiatry referral and support group involvement before discharge.
12. History may be not available immediately, but it plays a crucial role in further management and selection of antidote. Try to collect history from the ambulance crew, family and friends.

PARACETAMOL

- Most common drug overdose we encounter in our practice.
- Ingestions of greater than 7.5 g in an adult should be considered potentially toxic (150 mg/kg in healthy and 75 mg/kg in malnourished).
- It is well absorbed, with peak levels about four hours after an overdose.
- Ninety per cent of paracetamol is conjugated by the liver to nontoxic inactive compounds, which are renally excreted. About 5% excreted unchanged in urine and about 5% is oxidized by the P-450 mixed function oxidase enzyme to yield highly reactive toxic intermediates, which are detoxified by reduced glutathione. Toxicity occurs when the hepatic glutathione stores lose their ability to conjugate the toxic metabolite.
- Signs and symptoms:
  - Stage 1: 12–24 hours after ingestion; asymptomatic or mild GI symptoms
  - Stage 2: 24–72 hours; right upper quadrant pain, nausea and vomiting, liver enzymes begin to rise
  - Stage 3: 72–96 hours; maximal hepatic injury
  - Stage 4: either improvement or progression to acute liver necrosis with failure

- Management:
  - General supportive management as discussed above with specific importance to measurement of serum levels of paracetamol
  - Specific management:
    - **N-Acetylcysteine (NAC):** Effective if started within eight hours of ingestion. It acts by replenishing the depleted glutathione stores in the liver.
    - The **Rumack–Matthew** nomogram guides the use of NAC in acute overdoses.
    - The treatment line is based on a 4-hour half-life starting with a toxic 4-hour serum concentration of 150 mcg/mL.
    - This screening tool has a sensitivity of almost 100% when strictly applied.
    - NAC 150 mg/kg in 200 mL of 5% dextrose infused over 15 minutes, followed by 50 mg/kg in 500 mL 5% dextrose over 4 hours and 100 mg/kg in 1 L of 5% dextrose over 16 hours (total dose 300 mg/kg in 20 hours). Please refer to hospital protocol/TOXBASE for further guidance.
    - Maximum protective effect is time dependent. An ingestion-treatment interval of less than 10 hours gives the best results.
    - If ingestion time is unknown, or it is staggered, or the presentation is >15 hours from ingestion, treatment may help. Get advice from specialist centre.
    - Request liver function tests, and monitor urea and electrolyte levels. If the international normalised ratio (INR) is rising, continue NAC (100 mg/kg in 1 L of 5% dextrose over 16 hours).
    - Discuss with liver team. Do not hesitate to get help.

SALICYLATES

- Again, very common because of their availability, e.g. aspirin.
- Serious life-threatening toxicity is likely after ingestion of >7.5 g. Effects are dose related and potentially fatal.
- Causes uncoupling of oxidative phosphorylation, which leads to anaerobic metabolism and the production of lactate and heat.

- Clinical features:
  - Common – Tinnitus, vertigo, sweating, hyperventilation, pyrexia, vomiting, haematemesis. Watch for hyper-/hypoglycaemia
  - Rare – ↓GCS, seizures, hypotension, pulmonary oedema
  - Patients present with initial respiratory alkalosis due to stimulation of central respiratory centres and then develop metabolic alkalosis
- Management:
  - General management and investigations as described above
  - Treatment focused on increased excretion. This is achieved by
    - **Urine alkalinisation** – enhances salicylate elimination by trapping the ASA ion in the renal tubules and improving its removal. Achieved by giving 1.5 L of 1.26% sodium bicarbonate intravenously over three hours. Refer to hospital guidelines and TOXBASE in case of doubt.
    - **Haemodialysis** in more severe cases.
      - Discuss serious cases with the expert centre or National Poisons Information Service (NPIS).

SEDATIVES

- Benzodiazepines (BZD)
  - Overdose is common, but clinical features are not usually severe unless complicated by other central nervous system depressant drugs (alcohol), extremes of age, etc.
  - Clinical features include drowsiness, dysarthria, ataxia and nystagmus; however, agitation and confusion can occur.
  - General supportive management as above including activated charcoal.
  - Flumazenil may be used as a specific antidote (0.2 mg–1.0 mg intravenously given in 0.1-mg increments). Observe caution, as it is dangerous in BZD dependence and mixed poisoning with tricyclic antidepressants.
  - Reversal may be temporary as it is short acting and patient needs to be observed in a monitored environment.

- Barbiturates
    - Symptoms like BZD poisoning.
    - Treatment is supportive with attention to respiratory and cardio-vascular depression.
    - Activated charcoal and urine alkalinisation should be considered.
- Opioids
    - Treatment is again supportive with attention to respiratory depression and cardiovascular disturbance.
    - Naloxone may be used as an antidote (0.1 mg–0.4 mg). As it is short acting, reversal may be temporary.
    - Consider the risk of infection in intravenous drug users.

TRICYCLIC ANTIDEPRESSANTS

- Most common as they are prescribed to patients who are at greatest risk of suicide attempt.
- Account for up to one half of all overdose related adult intensive care admissions.
- Clinical features:
    - *Anticholinergic*: mydriasis, blurred vision, dry mouth, tachycardia, hyperpyrexia, urinary retention, decreased gut motility.
    - *CNS*: agitation, confusion, respiratory depression, seizures and coma.
    - *Cardiac*: wide QRS, PR, and QT intervals. Increased risk of arrhythmias. The best predictor is a QRS complex greater than 0.1 s or a prolonged QTc interval.
- Management:
    - General supportive management as above.
    - They are highly tissue bound and therefore serum concentrations do not correlate with toxicity and have little clinical value.
    - Patients require ECG monitoring during the initial period, monitor the QRS, QTc intervals and arrhythmias.
    - Serum alkalinisation with bicarbonate to achieve an arterial pH of 7.5 may reduce the risk of arrhythmias in patients with prolonged QRS/QTc interval. It also increases plasma protein binding and antagonizes the quinidine like effects on His-Purkinje system.
    - Seizures are best treated with diazepam/midazolam. Phenytoin is ineffective and may be dangerous.

Beta-blockers

- Most ingestions are benign. Those with cardiac disease are more at risk of complications.
- Two beta-blockers require special consideration:
    - Propranolol – causes sodium channel blockade – hypotension and bradycardia predominate and often refractory to standard resuscitation measures
    - Sotalol – causes potassium efflux blockade, monitor for Torsade's
- Management:
    - General supportive management as above
    - Prevent hypoglycaemia and hyperkalaemia
    - Specific antidotes:
        - *Glucagon* – 50 mcg/kg up to 10 mg, followed by infusion of 2–10 mg/hour.
        - High-dose insulin euglycaemic therapy (HIET)
            - Intravenous bolus of regular insulin at a dose of 1 unit/kg.
            - Monitor and maintain serum glucose with simultaneous dextrose infusion.
            - It is followed by a continuous infusion of insulin at a rate of 0.5–1 unit/kg/hour and dextrose at 0.5 g/kg/hour.
            - Serum glucose and potassium measurement every hour.
            - Increase insulin infusion by 0.5–1 unit/kg/hour every 60 minutes.
        - Consider *intralipid* if refractory to standard measures. Call for help as the situation is life threatening.
        - *Sodium bicarbonate* – to correct acidosis and treat arrhythmias; used as adjunct in QRS widening.
            - Discuss with tertiary centre and NPIS.

KEY LEARNING POINTS

- Manage via ABCDE.
- Get a history of the poison.
- General management is supportive.
- Contact TOXBASE or Poisons Information Service.

PART 8

MANAGEMENT

Pneumonia

JOSEPH HEROLD AND SHONDIPON K. LAHA

An 80-year-old gentleman is admitted to Intensive Care four days after a laparotomy. He is breathless and has a raised temperature. The decision was made to intubate the patient in order to correct his respiratory failure. After his intubation, his blood results are phoned by the lab: WCC of 13, raised urea of 8 mmol/L. The nursing staff inform you that the FiO_2 requirements are increasing and they are getting secretions when suctioning on ETT tube.

INTRODUCTION

Your patients usually present with pneumonia in four ways to a Critical Care Unit:

- Community-acquired pneumonia (CAP)
- Hospital-acquired pneumonia (HAP)
- Ventilator-associated pneumonia (VAP)
- Aspiration Pneumonia

The diagnostic criterion for each category of pneumonia is different. For each type, one must consider relevant patient factors.

General investigations that can be performed for patients suspected of pneumonia are

- Arterial blood gases (ABG)
- Full blood count (FBC)
- Urea and electrolytes (U&Es)
- Liver function test
- C-reactive protein (CRP)
- Chest X-ray
- One should also consider testing for atypical pneumonia, which would include urine samples for *Legionella* antigen

COMMUNITY-ACQUIRED PNEUMONIA (CAP)

Community-acquired pneumonia is defined currently by the British Thoracic Society as 'an acute illness with radiographic shadowing, which was at least segmental or present in more than one lobe and was not known to be previously present or due to other causes'. NICE has found that 5%–12% of adults presenting to their General Practice Doctors are diagnosed with a lower respiratory tract infection. Of these, 22%–42% are admitted in hospital with CAP. Of those that are admitted to the hospital, the mortality rate ranges from 5%–14%. The mortality rate for those that are admitted to the hospital and treated in Critical Care is about 30%, though 1%–10% of all cases are admitted to Critical Care.

TYPICAL ORGANISMS

- *Streptococcus pneumoniae*
- *Haemophilus influenzae*
- *Legionella* species
- *Staphylococcus aureus*

ATYPICALS

- *Mycoplasma pneumoniae*
- *Chlamydophila pneumoniae*
- *Chlamydia psittaci*
- *Coxiella burnetii*

Community-acquired pneumonia is graded using the CURB-65 score. This scoring should be done when the patient is first admitted to the hospital and CAP is suspected. The patient is scored 1 point for each of the following criteria:

- **C**onfusion (new onset of person, place, time)
- **R**aised **u**rea (>7 mmol/L)
- **R**espiratory rate (>30 breaths per min)
- **B**lood pressure (systolic less than 90 mmHg, or diastolic less than 60 mmHg)
- Age >**65**

The score a patient has can give a risk of death. Low risk is a score of 0–1 (<3%), intermediate is a score of 2 (3%–15%) and scores of 3–5 are high risk (>15%).

INVESTIGATIONS

Chest X-rays should be performed for these patients along with appropriate blood test. These would include white cell count (WCC), ABG, CRP, U&Es, blood and sputum cultures. You should send urine for *Pneumococcus* and *Legionella* antigens.

TREATMENT

Antibiotic treatment will vary from hospital to hospital; it is always best to consult local guidelines. In general with CURB-65 scores >3:

IV co-amoxiclav 1.2 g three times daily, and clarithromycin 500 mg twice a day,

Or if patient is allergic to penicillin:

IV cefuroxime 1.5 g three times a day, and clarithromycin 500 mg twice a day.

You should remember to review results of your blood and sputum cultures in order to adjust antibiotics to organisms grown. In general, you should expect these patients to complete a seven-day course of antibiotics and you should also be prepared to extend the course out to ten days for typical organisms. If the patient happens to have *Legionella*, staphylococcal, or Gram-negative enteric bacteria, the course could be up to 21 days depending on the patient and signs of improvement. Oxygen therapy should be titrated with use of ABGs. Non-invasive ventilation has shown use only if there is acute exacerbation of COPD.

HOSPITAL-ACQUIRED PNEUMONIA (HAP)

Hospital-acquired pneumonia occurs if a patient develops new symptoms after 48 hours in the hospital. You must also rule out hospital-acquired infections if that patient has been recently discharged from the hospital (if less than ten days in length). If patients are admitted from long-term care facilities, then you must rule out hospital bacteria. Local guidance from the hospital microbiologist should be taken to target antibiotic therapy appropriately for each specific region. In critical care settings, one must also remember secondary pneumonia, as these may not be the primary admission diagnosis, for example aspiration pneumonia.

It is common to find patients that have been admitted to Critical Care units that will have underlying chest infections whether this be CAP, HAP or aspiration. The patients that are at risk for aspiration are those that have received CPR, admitted with low consciousness level, and patients with swallowing difficulties. Diagnosis of aspiration is if the patient presents with risk factors and radiologic evidence of infiltrates suggestive of aspiration.

Common organisms causing HAP include

- *Escherichia coli*
- *Klebsiella pneumoniae*

- *Pseudomonas aeruginosa*
- *Acinetobacter* species
- *Staphylococcus aureus* including methicillin-resistant *S. aureus* (MRSA)

Less common organisms in HAP include

- *Streptococci viridans*
- Coagulase-negative *Staphylococci*
- *Neisseria* species
- *Corynebacterium* species

TREATMENT OF HAP

Antibiotic treatment again will vary from hospital to hospital and region. There is normally a microbiology-led pathway for treatment. Usual regimes include the following.

If early onset of HAP occurs (admission <5 days), then consider oral antibiotics; if patient is unable to ingest tablets, then consider intravenous antibiotics. The most commonly used medications are tazobactam/piperacillin combinations (4.5 g three times a day depending on renal function). If the patient is allergic to penicillin, intravenous cephalosporins with metronidazole can be considered.

ASPIRATION PNEUMONIA

Common organisms include

- *Streptococcus pneumoniae*
- *Staphylococcus aureus*
- *Haemophilus influenza*
- *Enterobacteriaceae*
- *Pseudomonas aeruginosa*

VENTILATOR-ASSOCIATED PNEUMONIA (VAP)

The quoted incidence of VAP varies greatly; a 2012 article published in the *British Medical Journal* reported incidence as high as 27%. This is usually defined as pneumonia in a patient that has been intubated and ventilated currently or within 48 hours post intubation (BMJ, 2012). VAPs increase patient mortality up to 30% in critical care settings, as well as the number of days the patient requires the ventilator.

The organisms that are typically seen in early onset VAPs are similar to those found in AP. Organisms in late-onset VAPs (>4 days admission) are more likely to be Gram-positive organisms, with *Staphylococcus aureus*, *Pseudomonas*, and *Klebsiella* commonly isolated.

DIAGNOSIS

Clinical findings and the use of scoring systems are the best at attempting to diagnose VAP. Different hospitals use different criteria but they tend to be based on the score below.

THE CLINICAL PULMONARY INFECTION SCORE (CPIS) FOR VAP

Score	0	1	2
Temperature (°C)	36.5–37.9	38.0–38.9	<36.5 or >39.0
White blood cell count 10^9/litre	4.0–11.0	<4 or >11	>11
Tracheal secretions		+	++/purulent
PaO_2/FiO_2 ratio (mmHg)	>240 or ARDS	<240 and no ARDS	
Radiology	No infiltrate	Diffuse/patchy infiltrate	Localized infiltrate
Tracheal aspirate culture	Negative		Positive

The use of sputum cultures is important to mention in the diagnosis of VAP, as there are a number of ways cultures can be obtained. The first is the use of non-directed broncho-alveolar lavage in which 10 mL of saline is introduced into the trachea via either the endotracheal tube or tracheostomy and then suctioned out in an aseptic manner. The second is blind brachial sampling in which suction catheters are directed into the relevant lobes without the use of bronchoscopy. The last is using a bronchoscope to directly visualise the main bronchi and to insure that samples are taken from the appropriate locations. Unfortunately, this method is time consuming and the most invasive.

PREVENTION OF VAP

Because of the increase in patient mortality, ventilator days and stay in Critical Care, every effort should be made to prevent VAP. Typical prevention bundles will vary between hospitals but should include the following:

- Reviewing of patients sedation, considering sedation holidays
- Accessing patients for weaning and extubation daily
- Nursing the patient in 30° head up if able
- Use of subglottic endotracheal tubes
- Chlorhexidine mouth care and good dental hygiene (completed four times a day)

Other measures may be included to help reduce the risk of VAP:

- Meticulous hand hygiene practices
- Maintaining adequate cuff pressure
- Changing of ventilator circuits (at least twice weekly)

The best method is still to avoid intubation if possible.

TREATMENT

Antibiotics should be used according to local guidelines. If treating early onset VAP, treat as one would treat CAP using co-amoxiclav, for example. If treating a later onset of VAP, tazobactam/piperacillin or ciprofloxacin are commonly used. The common course of antibiotics for VAP is five days but may be extended to 7–10 depending on the patient. Antibiotics will need to be adjusted according to organisms found on culture. Intensive care patients are more likely to encounter rarer drug-resistant organisms so they should be managed with microbiology input from an early stage.

WHAT DO YOU DO IN RESPONSE TO THE NURSE'S QUESTION?

There are several signs that the patient is likely to have HAP. He has a temperature, raised white cell count, increasing respiratory tract secretions and is hypoxic. He should be placed on antibiotics according to local guidelines.

KEY LEARNING POINTS

- Early recognition of pneumonia is key.
- Pneumonias can be split into three groups.
- Antibiotics are given according to local protocol as soon as a diagnosis is made.

FURTHER READING

British Thoracic Society. *BTS Guidelines for the Management of Community Acquired Pneumonia in Adults.* British Thoracic Society, London, July 2009.

British Thoracic Society. *Annotated BTS Guideline for the Management of CAP in Adults 2015.* British Thoracic Society, London, January 2015, www .brit-thoracic.org.uk/standards-of-care/guidelines/bts-guidelines-for-the -management-of-community-acquired-pneumonia-in-adults-update-2009 /annotated-bts-guideline-for-the-management-of-cap-in-adults-2015 (accessed 10 November 2017).

Hunter, John D. "Ventilator Associated Pneumonia." *The BMJ 344* (May 2012): e3325. www.bmj.com/content/bmj/344/bmj.e3325.full.pdf (accessed 10 November 2017).

Kalil, Andre C., Mark L. Metersky, Michael Klompas, John Muscedere, Daniel A. Sweeney, Lucy B. Palmer, Lena M. Napolitano, Naomi P. O'Grady, John G. Bartlett, Jordi Carratalà, Ali A. El Solh, Santiago Ewig, Paul D. Fey, Thomas M. File, Jr., Marcos I. Restrepo, Jason A. Roberts, Grant W. Waterer, Peggy Cruse, Shandra L. Knight, and Jan L. Brozek. "Management of Adults with Hospital-Acquired and Ventilator-Associated Pneumonia: 2016 Clinical Practice Guidelines by the Infectious Diseases Society of America and the American Thoracic Society." *Clinical Infectious Diseases 63,* no. 5 (September 2016): e61–e111, www.thoracic.org/statements/resources/tb-opi/hap -vap-guidelines-2016.pdf (accessed 10 November 2017).

National Institute of Health and Care Excellence, *Pneumonia in Adults: Diagnosis and Management,* Clinical Guideline CG191, National Institute of Health and Care Excellence, Manchester, December 2014, www.nice.org.uk/guidance/cg191 (accessed 10 November 2017).

Acute severe asthma

CARL GROVES AND GOVINDAN RAGHURAMAN

You are on-call for ICU and receive a bleep from the Emergency Department (ED): a 29-year-old female is currently in the Resuscitation room. She is short of breath, wheezy and unable to complete full sentences. Initial management for asthma has been given but she is not responding so they have called for your assistance.

WHAT CAUSES ASTHMA?

According to Asthma UK, 5.4 million people are receiving treatment for asthma; on average, three people per day die from the disease. Asthma is characterised by reversible airway obstruction resulting from bronchial smooth muscle hypersensitivity, airway inflammation and increased mucosal secretions. Symptoms range from mild cough and wheeze to life-threatening airway obstruction and subsequent respiratory failure.

Precipitants may include

- Exposure to allergen, e.g. pollens, animals, cigarette smoke
- Upper or lower respiratory tract infection
- Poor compliance with asthma treatments
- Cold air or exercise
- Emotional stress

DIAGNOSIS OF ACUTE SEVERE ASTHMA

Patients typically present with wheeze, breathlessness and cough. Symptoms can develop over minutes, hours or days. The features of acute severe, life-threatening and near-fatal asthma are shown below (Table 38.1).

The history should be focused and aim to identify features that may predict rapid progression or deterioration:

- Previous near-fatal asthma requiring ventilation
- Previous hospital admissions
- Three or more asthma medications
- 'Brittle' asthma
- Non-compliance with treatment/appointments

Table 38.1 Features of severe asthma

Acute severe asthma	Life threatening asthma	Near fatal asthma
PEF 35%–50% best/ predicted RR 25/min HR >110/min Inability to complete sentences in one breath	Altered conscious level PEF <33% Exhaustion SpO$_2$ <92% PaO$_2$ <8 kPa, regardless of FiO$_2$ Low pH/High [H+] Arrhythmia Hypotension Normal PaCO$_2$ Cyanosis Silent chest Poor respiratory effort Or acute severe asthma not responding to treatment	Raised PaCO$_2$ Requiring mechanical ventilation with raised inflation pressures

Remember to consider other important differential diagnoses:

- Pneumothorax – any tracheal deviation/lateralising signs?
- Upper airway obstruction – inspiratory stridor rather than expiratory wheeze
- Pneumonia/chest infection – focal rather than general wheeze, purulent sputum

INVESTIGATIONS

PEAK EXPIRATORY FLOW (PEF) OR FEV1

Allows measurement of airway calibre and assessment of severity and response to treatment. Most useful when compared to patients normal PEF as a percentage; however, if this is not known, the predicted value can be used.

PULSE OXIMETRY

Patients with acute severe asthma can be, but are not always, hypoxaemic. Good oxygen saturation levels do not mean they do not have severe asthma. The aim of oxygen therapy is to maintain saturations of 94%–98%. This will guide the need for an ABG.

ARTERIAL BLOOD GASES (ABGS)

Patients with any features of life-threatening asthma or if oxygen saturations are <92% (on air or oxygen) require an ABG measurement. They should also be taken on any patients with severe asthma who are not responding to initial treatment. Saturations of less than 92% are associated with a risk of developing hypercapnia.

It may be useful to insert an arterial line to facilitate regular ABG sampling given that the patient is in the appropriate environment.

Beware the patient with a normal $PaCO_2$ as this can be a sign they are starting to tire; an asthmatic is often tachypnoeic, so their $PaCO_2$ should be low. A raised arterial carbon dioxide (CO_2) level suggests imminent danger of respiratory/cardiac arrest.

Indications for chest X-ray are as follows:

- Suspected pneumothorax or pneumomediatstinum
- Suspected consolidation
- Life-threatening asthma
- Failure to respond to treatment satisfactorily
- Requirement for ventilation

MANAGEMENT

You arrive in ED. The patient is still unable to talk in full sentences. She has received salbutamol and ipratropium nebulisers. Her heart rate is 140 bpm, and respiratory rate is 30 breaths/min. SpO_2 is 93% on 15 L O_2 using a mask with a reservoir bag.

Remember your ABCs.

1. Make sure the airway is patent.
2. Give 100% oxygen initially.
3. Obtain IV access.
4. Ensure full monitoring including pulse oximetry, three-lead ECG monitoring.

INITIAL TREATMENT

OXYGEN

- Patients with acute severe asthma are hypoxaemic; oxygen should be delivered at flow rates to maintain SpO_2 of 94%–98%.
- All nebulisers should be driven with oxygen and not air.

BETA-2 AGONIST BRONCHODILATOR

- Salbutamol 5 mg nebulisers can be given every 15–30 min, as a first-line treatment.
- Can be continuously nebulised if equipment available at 5–10 mg/hr is poorly responsive to initial treatment.
- Intravenous salbutamol can be given in ventilated patients or those in extremis but has not been shown to be more effective than nebulisers. IV salbutamol is useful when nebulisers cannot be used reliably.
- Dose initially 5 mcg/minute peripherally (range 3–20 mcg/minute).

IPRATROPIUM BROMIDE

- Anti-cholinergic, which is very effective when used in combination with β_2-agonists when compared with β_2-agonists alone
- Nebulised solution 0.5 mg every 4–6 hours

STEROIDS

- Reduces mortality, relapses and reduces β_2-agonist requirements. The earlier they are given, the better the outcome.
- There is no evidence that IV steroids are any more effective than oral formulations.
- Prednisolone 40 mg daily or hydrocortisone 100 mg every six hours. This should be continued for five days.

INTRAVENOUS FLUIDS

- There are no controlled trials that suggest the benefit of fluids in asthma; however, patients may require rehydration or correction of hypokalaemia.

TREATMENT INITIATED AFTER CONSULTATION WITH SENIOR STAFF

The following treatments can be considered if there is a poor response to the above treatments.

MAGNESIUM SULPHATE

- IV magnesium sulphate peripherally 1.2–2 g infusion over 20 minutes (as recommended by the BTS guidelines). May need to give more – often up to 5 g

Aminophylline infusion

- Generally not more effective than standard treatment
- IV 5 mg/kg loading dose over 20 minutes (omit if on oral theophyllines)
- Followed by infusion 0.5–0.7 mg/kg/hr

The following can be considered in extremis or when having difficulty with mechanical ventilation.

Adrenaline

- Can be given as bolus 1 mL 1:10,000 or as infusion. Only to be used if patient in extremis after failure of above treatment
- High risk of arrhythmias
- Can also be given subcutaneously or via endotracheal tube

Anaesthetic inhalational agents

- If equipment is available. Can be used if all other treatments fail. Sevoflurane is the preferred volatile agent since it is a non-irritant to airways.

Ketamine

- A sedative/anaesthetic agent given as bolus or infusion particularly if intubation required

VENTILATION

Non-invasive

- Limited evidence but may be beneficial in some patients.
- Unlikely to help in patients who are tired or with raised CO_2 levels.
- More RCTs needed to identify patients who would benefit.

INVASIVE

- Patients with severe bronchospasm are often very difficult to ventilate.
- Only small tidal volumes may be possible due to high airway pressures.
- Ventilate with low or no PEEP (as these patients may have high 'autoPEEP').
- A low respiratory rate with prolonged expiratory phase may be needed with I:E ratios of 1:3, 1:4 or higher.
- These ventilatory measures may cause high $PaCO_2$, which should be tolerated (permissive hypercapnia).
- Patients may need to be heavily sedated or paralysed.
- 'Gas trapping' due to bronchospasm; gas finds it difficult to leave the alveoli. This leads to progressively higher airway pressures with decreasing tidal volumes and increased risk of pneumothorax. Gas trapping can be countered by allowing adequate expiratory time between breaths. If a patient has severe gas trapping, their tidal volumes will be low, and intrathoracic pressure high. This can cause cardiovascular collapse or respiratory compromise. Disconnecting the ventilator from the endotracheal tube is often useful in this emergency.

Treatments not clinically recommended:

- Antibiotics – Usually viral trigger, therefore antibiotics not needed unless purulent sputum or other signs of infection
- Heliox – No evidence of efficacy in asthmatic patients
- Leukotriene receptor antagonists – Insufficient evidence for use in acute exacerbation

WHAT IS THE PROGNOSIS OF ASTHMA AND HOW DO I PREVENT IT?

Asthma is a chronic condition and it will need regular treatment to prevent exacerbation. Once the patient is stable post discharge from ICU, it is a good opportunity to review the patient's asthma treatment, compliance with medication and aid the patient in removing precipitants where possible. Patients with brittle asthma should be referred to asthma specialists for further management. Currently significant advancements have been made in providing stability for such patients through advent of newer biologic treatments.

KEY LEARNING POINTS

- Asthma can kill; early management is essential.
- A silent chest, rising CO_2 or hypoxia are warning signs that patient may need intubation.
- Call for senior help if intubating/ventilating an asthmatic patient.

FURTHER READING

British Thoracic Society/Scottish Intercollegiate Guidelines Network. "BTS/SIGN British Guideline on the Management of Asthma: A National Clinical Guideline." SIGN 153, September 2016.

Stanley, David, and William Tunnicliffe. "Management of Life-Threatening Asthma in Adults." *Continuing Education in Anaesthesia Critical Care & Pain* 8, no. 3 (June 2008): 95–99.

The COPD patient in intensive care

DANIEL PARK

'Mr Evans was admitted breathless with COPD overnight but now he looks worse than ever despite treatment: do you think he needs to go on a ventilator?'

INTRODUCTION

Chronic obstructive pulmonary disease (COPD) is a common lung condition characterised by shortness of breath, chronic cough, wheeze and regular sputum production. The main risk factor for the development of COPD is tobacco smoking, but it can also be caused by air pollution or industrial exposures. COPD is believed to affect approximately 5% of the global population, and causes millions of deaths worldwide.

Acute exacerbations of COPD are a frequent cause of admission to the hospital, and of subsequent referral to critical care. There are many people living in the community with a level of respiratory function that is adequate for them to manage day-to-day, but that when put under additional strain (most often due to a respiratory tract infection) rapidly causes worsening symptoms and may lead to decompensated respiratory failure requiring ventilator support.

The sick patient with COPD requires appropriate initial assessment and accurate diagnosis. Is this an acute exacerbation of COPD or is there consolidation on the chest X-ray indicating pneumonia? Subsequently, optimal medical management should be given in the correct setting within your institution. Close monitoring for signs of deterioration and need for an escalation of therapy is important, in association with an early decision as to whether such escalation is appropriate.

PHARMACOLOGICAL MANAGEMENT OF AN EXACERBATION OF COPD

First line pharmacological therapy for an exacerbation of COPD consists of

- Acute bronchodilator therapy
- Controlled oxygen therapy
- Oral steroids (30 mg prednisolone OD for 7–14 days)
- Antibiotic therapy as per local guidelines

Bronchodilator therapy is best delivered to patients with a significant exacerbation of COPD via a nebuliser – often they are too breathless to be able to use anything else. Both a beta-2 agonist (e.g. salbutamol) and anti-muscarinic (e.g. ipratropium bromide) should be offered. Patients with COPD exacerbations sufficiently severe as to bring them to hospital should generally have their nebulisers driven by air – over-oxygenation (i.e. elevating a patient's blood level of oxygen above their normal value) can exacerbate hypercapnia by both worsening VQ mismatch and blunting the hypoxic drive to breathe.

Oxygen delivery should therefore be tightly controlled in this patient group. Hypoxia is life threatening and should be avoided at all costs;

however, hypercapnia from over-provision of oxygen can increase the need for ventilator support. In the first instance, an oxygen saturation of 88%–92% or PaO$_2$ of 8 kPa is targeted, (although this may require subsequent modification depending on the individual response.) The use of fixed performance interfaces (e.g. a Venturi mask) for oxygen delivery can be helpful by reliably providing the chosen inspired percentage of oxygen irrespective of any variation in the patient's breathing over time.

Antibiotics should be given as per your local guidelines. Remember antibiotics suggested for an acute exacerbation of COPD are likely to be different to those for community-acquired pneumonia.

VENTILATOR SUPPORT FOR PATIENTS WITH COPD

Some patients will require ventilator support despite the best medical management. This can be provided using a non-invasive or invasive approach, although neither is provided without considerable discomfort to the patient. Consideration should always be given as to whether the patient is an appropriate candidate, taking into account not just their acute physiological condition, but also the severity of their underlying lung disease, co-morbidities, performance status, and most importantly, the patient's own wishes for the type of treatment they would like to receive. Palliation of symptoms is sometimes an appropriate course. Decisions as to the resuscitation status for the patient and any ceiling of therapy should be made and discussed prior to embarking on the provision of ventilator support, and reviewed regularly thereafter.

NON-INVASIVE VENTILATION FOR PATIENTS WITH COPD

Non-invasive ventilation (NIV) refers to ventilator support, which is provided without the need for an endotracheal tube or tracheostomy. Its use has increased dramatically in the last three decades. NIV decreases the work of breathing and improves gas exchange and minute ventilation. This is not a treatment for the underlying lung pathology of itself, but supports the patient's respiratory system whilst they recover. It has proved particularly effective for the patient with COPD. The ventilator provides a lower level of support in expiration (expiratory positive airway pressure or EPAP) and senses when the patient breathes in to provide a higher level of support (inspiratory positive airway pressure or IPAP). A back-up rate of machine delivered breaths can also be set.

NIV has the major advantage of avoiding the many complications of invasive ventilation; this is particularly important in an often frail and elderly patient suffering from an acute exacerbation of COPD. However, there are a number of contraindications to its use, which include the following:

- Recent facial/upper airway surgery
- Facial abnormalities such as burns or trauma
- Vomiting
- Inability to protect the airway
- Confusion/agitation
- Recent upper gastrointestinal surgery
- Copious respiratory secretions
- Untreated pneumothorax – should generally be drained prior to NIV
- Base-of-skull fracture

Whether these factors preclude the use of NIV entirely will depend on the individual case, and factors such as whether NIV is the ceiling of therapy, and the setting in which NIV is to be provided.

NIV usually works pretty quickly if it is going to work at all – improvement should be seen within the first hour of therapy. Failure is evidenced by worsening respiratory rate, deteriorating gas exchange, tiring/distressed patient and ultimately a reducing conscious level.

WHERE SHOULD NIV BE DELIVERED?

Different institutions provide NIV for patients with COPD in different types of units and with different sets of physicians directing therapy. Provision may be on a respiratory ward or respiratory/medical high dependency area under the care of respiratory or general medical physicians, or on a high dependency/intensive care unit under the care of intensivists. Patients cared for on a respiratory ward should have only single organ failure, and this setting is better suited to those who are more stable, with less deranged physiology, and to those for whom NIV is an agreed ceiling of therapy. Conversely, the more unstable patients – particularly those for whom invasive ventilation is to be offered in the event of failure of NIV – are generally better looked after in higher care areas. Patients proceeding with NIV despite a relative contraindication merit closer monitoring than may be available on a general ward. Patients requiring a significant degree of oxygenation during their NIV therapy will also generally need a higher care area. NIV, as provided on most respiratory wards, uses ventilators, which entrain oxygen from a flow meter into the ventilator circuit – this arrangement offers much lower and more variable fractions of inspired oxygen than the ventilators used on a critical care unit, usually reaching 50% at best. Critical care ventilators draw their oxygen directly from the pressurised wall supply, and can reliably deliver up to 100% through an NIV facemask.

HOW IS NIV PROVIDED?

NIV can be a frightening experience for an already unwell and distressed patient. Initial settings should be gentle, and gradually titrated upwards until the desired degree of support is reached. An interface should be chosen to minimise leaks and maximise patient comfort. Reassurance should be provided to the patient throughout.

Often more or less continuous ventilator support is required initially – with breaks for comfort or meals as tolerated. Once the patient's condition has stabilised, the therapy can be weaned. There is no clear evidence as to how this is best done – most units will use a pragmatic approach of lengthening the amount of time without support and checking to ensure the patient is comfortable and there is no physiological derangement. Ventilation is always more compromised at night even in the stable patient with COPD, and NIV should be weaned in the daytime first.

INVASIVE VENTILATION FOR PATIENTS WITH COPD

The majority of patients with COPD needing ventilator support will be able to be treated with NIV; however, a minority will require intubation and invasive mechanical ventilation because NIV failed, was contraindicated or just not tolerated. Intensivists have traditionally been seen as reluctant to offer such therapy – worried that patients with COPD will not 'get off the ventilator' and that their prognosis is uniformly dreadful. More recently, this attitude is changing – whilst many patients with COPD requiring intubation do have a poor prognosis, when appropriately selected this is not worse than other groups requiring level III care. Careful consideration needs to be made of each case, and the risks and benefits discussed with the patient and/or their family. A scoring system is available to help try to predict six-month mortality (see 'Further Reading'). Amongst the most important considerations are patient performance status, age, degree of physiological derangement, days since hospital admission and nutritional status.

COPD patients in critical care can behave very variably, reflecting the heterogeneity of the underlying disease. Some patients need only a short period of invasive ventilation – enough to allow their respiratory musculature to rest and recover whilst the worst of their exacerbation is treated, or to correct their hypercapnia and restore their conscious level. Others have a much stormier course. Some patients have very marked bronchospasm, and behave just like an asthmatic – indeed many of those labelled with 'COPD' probably have overlapping conditions. In these individuals, anything that might worsen it further should be avoided. Intubation itself may prompt bronchospasm, and should only be carried out under appropriate anaesthesia. During intubation and subsequent sedation, drugs that may promote histamine release are best avoided, e.g. morphine, atracurium. The use of an agent (e.g. ketamine) with bronchodilatory effects for induction of anaesthesia may be helpful. Paralysis may be necessary. Once placed on a ventilator, the patient with COPD may require high positive inspiratory pressures, which can cause cardiovascular instability by restricting venous return. This is a particular problem if the patient is not fully fluid resuscitated prior to intubation. Positive pressure ventilation at any level, but especially if high inflation pressures are used, puts the COPD patient at particular risk of the development of a pneumothorax, which may rapidly increase 'tension'. This is a life-threatening emergency, which if not identified and treated immediately, will lead to cardiopulmonary arrest.

The 'obstructive' part of COPD describes the difficulty such patients have with lung emptying (something which can be exacerbated by over-enthusiastic mechanical ventilation). Ventilator settings need to be chosen that minimise peak pressures, and offer a prolonged expiratory time, which prevents a new breath being taken before the last has been fully expired. An I:E ratio of 1:3 or higher may be needed to ensure that this 'breath stacking' does not occur.

If the patient is attempting to breathe spontaneously, care must be taken to ensure that such breaths are effectively triggering the ventilator. Air trapping due to delayed lung emptying can lead to the generation of 'intrinsic PEEP' (PEEPi). This needs to be overcome by the patient before they can generate sufficient pressure change to trigger support for inspiration from the ventilator. Unsupported attempts at breathing add considerably to the patient's workload and difficulties in synchronising with the ventilator. PEEPi can be offset by the judicious use of extrinsic PEEP ventilator settings.

COPD patients in critical care should continue to receive bronchodilator therapy, corticosteroids and appropriate antibiotics. Bronchodilators can be provided through in-line nebulisers placed in the ventilator circuit.

Alternatively, salbutamol can be given intravenously, and titrated to effect. Intravenous aminophylline can also be considered, although evidence for its efficacy in this situation is limited, and has significant side effects including tachycardia and nausea. Those patients who have persistent bronchospasm may benefit from a ketamine infusion or even the use of a volatile anaesthetic agent (e.g. sevoflurane). Anaesthetic gases have to be given either with the use of an anaesthetic machine or using a scavenging system for the ventilator waste gases, otherwise staff members are exposed to the drug.

Patients with COPD are a group particularly likely to benefit from early extubation to NIV therapy. This has the advantage of limiting the complications of invasive ventilation (including through reducing exposure to sedation and other medications, limiting reduction in muscle loss from immobility, improving nutrition, allowing better communication and so on), whilst continuing to provide ventilator support as required. Evidence available at present suggests that early extubation to NIV of COPD patients in particular improves critical care length of stay and mortality.

WHAT ABOUT MR EVANS?

Go and see Mr Evans – has he been correctly diagnosed and optimally treated? If so and his condition is continuing to deteriorate, he is indeed likely to require ventilator support. Can this be provided non-invasively? Where can this be done in your institution? Ask yourself: would he be an appropriate candidate for intubation and mechanical ventilation? Is this what *he* wants?

KEY LEARNING POINTS

In patients with COPD:
- NIV should be considered for initial ventilator support in the absence of contraindications.
- Breath stacking, the failure to effectively trigger support from the ventilator and tension pneumothorax can complicate invasive ventilation.
- Early extubation to NIV reduces ICU length of stay and mortality.

FURTHER READING

Burns, Karen E.A., Maureen O. Meade, Azra Premji, and Neill K.J. Adhikari. "Noninvasive Positive-Pressure Ventilation as a Weaning Strategy for Intubated Adults with Respiratory Failure." *Cochrane Database of Systematic Reviews*, no. 12 (December 2013), Article No. CD004127.

National Institute of Health and Care Excellence. "Chronic Obstructive Pulmonary Disease in Over 16s: Diagnosis and Management." Clinical Guideline CG101, National Institute for Health and Care Excellence, Manchester, June 2010 (updated April 2016). www.nice.org.uk/guidance /cg101 (accessed 3 December 2016).

Wildman, Martin J., Colin Sanderson, Jayne Groves, Barnaby C. Reeves, Jon G. Ayres, David A. Harrison, Duncan Young, and Kathryn M. Rowan. "Predicting Mortality for Patients with Exacerbations of COPD and Asthma in the COPD and Asthma Outcome Study (CAOS)." *QJM: An International Journal of Medicine* 102, no. 6 (June 2009): 389–399.

40

Acute respiratory distress syndrome

RICHARD BENSON AND CRAIG SPENCER

A 42-year-old female presents to the emergency department with a 48-hour history of worsening shortness of breath, non-productive cough, high temperatures and lethargy. Her past medical history includes asthma.

On review she has a high respiratory rate of 35, oxygen saturations of 90% on 15 L via a reservoir bag, and a heart rate of 140 BPM.

An arterial blood gas reveals a PaO_2 of 6.5 kPa and a $PaCO_2$ of 7 kPa with a pH of 7.25. An initial chest X-ray reveals bilateral opacities.

She is intubated and transferred to the intensive care unit with a provisional diagnosis of ARDS.

WHAT IS ARDS?

Acute respiratory distress syndrome (ARDS) is a severe form of respiratory failure and is often a result of severe physiological insult. Over the last few years, not only has its definition changed but also its treatment, and this remains an evolving area.

ARDS is characterised by non-cardiogenic pulmonary oedema. It leads to diffuse alveolar and interstitial lung oedema, loss of surfactant and alveolar flooding with a proteinaceous exudate containing macrophages and neutrophils. This results in stiff, noncompliant lungs and hypoxaemia. The pathophysiology of the condition is complex and believed to be immunologically mediated by cytokines causing an inflammatory cascade and loss of capillary integrity. After 7–10 days, a fibro-proliferative stage develops resulting in pulmonary fibrosis.

There should be a known precipitant for ARDS, initiating the inflammatory response causing lung injury. This may be a direct pulmonary cause such as pneumonia, contusion, aspiration or smoke inhalation. Extra-pulmonary/systemic causes include sepsis, trauma, massive transfusion and pancreatitis.

Patients present with respiratory distress, including tachypnoea and cyanosis, in conjunction with the signs of the precipitating condition.

DIAGNOSIS

In 2013, the Berlin definition was formed which removed the sub-classification of Acute Lung Injury. Its main components are

- Acute (onset less than one week)
- Bilateral opacities on chest imaging (CT or CXR) not explained by other lung pathology

- Respiratory failure not explained by heart failure or fluid overload
- PaO_2/FiO_2 (PF) ratio < 300 mmHg (< 40 kPa) with a minimum of 5 cmH$_2$O of PEEP

ARDS can be further classified by severity based on the PaO_2/FiO_2 ratio:

- Mild ARDS: 201–300 mmHg (≤ 39.9 kPa)
- Moderate ARDS: 101–200 mmHg (≤ 26.6 kPa)
- Severe ARDS: ≤ 100 mmHg (≤ 13.3 kPa)

TREATMENT

Treatment is directed to treating the precipitating cause of ARDS. Strategies for treatment of ARDS can initially appear numerous and complex but they can be simplified by dividing them into ventilation strategies, patients positioning, pharmacological options and extra corporeal treatments.

VENTILATION STRATEGIES

- Intubation and ventilation is the mainstay of supportive therapy. Aims focus on avoidance of hypoxia, avoidance of excessive hypercapnia and avoidance of ventilator-associated pneumonia.
- The ARDSNet paper of 2000 was a landmark multicentre randomised controlled trial (RCT), which demonstrated a significant reduction in mortality for a tidal volume of 6 mL/kg versus 12 mL/kg (Brower et al., 2000). Tidal volume is based on Ideal Body Weight, which is best calculated using the patient's height. This trial also led to the introduction of permissive hypercapnia and plateau pressures of less than 30 cmH$_2$O.
- *Permissive hypercapnia*. With low tidal volumes, hypercapnia is almost inevitable. A respiratory acidosis is usually tolerated down to around pH 7.2. Below this level, options include increasing respiratory rate (risk of reducing the expiratory time and 'breath stacking'), IV sodium bicarbonate (may cause intracellular acidosis) or relaxing the tidal volume limit to 7 or 8 mL/Kg.
- *Open lung ventilation*. Positive End Expiratory Pressure (PEEP) is used to keep recruited alveoli open, avoid atelectrauma and improve

oxygenation. In ARDS, the lung is not homogenous and excessive PEEP risks overdistention in less affected parts, as well as cardiovascular effects such as reduced venous return with high intra-thoracic pressure. Choosing the right level of PEEP is difficult; a commonly used scale of 5–20 cm of PEEP that increases with FiO_2 is a good starting point.

- *Inverse ratio ventilation.* A physiological I:E ratio (Inspiratory/Expiratory time ratio) is 1:2 to allow time for passive expiration of CO_2. At a high FiO_2, increasing the inspiratory time or even reversing the ratio from 1:2 to 2:1 gives extra time for inspiratory flow to redistribute to difficult-to-recruit alveoli. It may increase hypercapnia by reducing time for passive CO_2 excretion.

- *Airway Pressure Release Ventilation (APRV).* APRV utilises an inverse ratio ventilator strategy with unrestricted spontaneous ventilation over the top of the two levels of PEEP set. PEEP high is set much longer than PEEP low, which often results in a degree of autoPEEP. Initial settings may be: PEEP high 25, PEEP low 0–5, time in PEEP high 6 seconds, time in PEEP low 1 second. This mode may improve ventilation due to alveolar recruitment but it does risk excessive tidal volumes and increases the amount of work on the right ventricle.

- *High Frequency Oscillation Ventilation (HFOV).* Oscillation uses a specialised ventilator to deliver small tidal volumes (around 100 mL) at very high respiratory rates (3–15 cycles/second). Despite initial optimism, it is now virtually obsolete following the early termination of a multicentre RCT of 548 patients (OSCILLATE), which showed a significant increase in mortality with HFOV versus low tidal volume controlled ventilation (Ferguson et al., 2013).

POSITIONING

PRONE VENTILATION

The prone position offers better ventilation/perfusion matching and less lung base compression by the abdomen. PROSEVA was a multicentre RCT published in 2013, which showed a significant reduction of 16% versus 32.8% in mortality with better oxygenation and less ventilator days (Guérin et al. 2013).

The way in which prone positioning is undertaken is likely to be dependent on the unit in which you work.

The chest and pelvis should be supported to allow abdominal movement with ventilation. Risks include displacement of the airway and lines, facial pressure sores and eye injuries. Benefits improve with early proning (<36 hours of onset) and longer daily proning episodes (16–20 hours).

PHARMACOLOGICAL APPROACHES

SEDATION

Patients may need to be heavily sedated to tolerate relatively un-physiological ventilation strategies of noncompliant lungs, especially in the prone position. It may be necessary to abolish all patient effort in the early stages. Sedation is best titrated to a prescribed sedation score (e.g. Richmond Agitation-Sedation Score – RASS scale). As lung mechanics improve, daily sedation holds may enable spontaneous patient effort.

MUSCLE RELAXANTS

Atracurium and cis-atracurium are the two drugs you are likely to come across, and can be given by a bolus or infusion. They can be beneficial for preventing ventilator asynchrony and may lead to more ventilator free days but care should be taken to ensure the patient is completely sedated.

STEROIDS

Multiple trials have addressed whether the use of steroids may be beneficial particularly in reducing the later fibro-proliferative stage of ARDS between 7 and 14 days post-onset. Evidence is mixed, as is practice, though most centres do not use routinely.

PULMONARY VASODILATORS

When inhaled at concentrations up to 40 ppm, nitric oxide crosses the alveoli in ventilated parts of the lung causing local vasodilation and improved ventilation-perfusion matching and oxygenation. Like proning, there are responders and non-responders. Only rarely used as a rescue therapy, no mortality benefit has been proven.

INTRAVENOUS FLUID

Increased extravascular lung water is associated with increased mortality and prolonged respiratory weaning. A protocol of restrictive fluid administration regime including the use of diuretics, aiming for an even fluid balance at seven days post onset is associated with improved oxygenation and reduced time on a ventilator (but not mortality), without increasing the need for renal replacement therapy. Haemofiltration or haemodialysis may be considered for fluid removal in patients who are oliguric or anuric as part of multi-organ failure, and this may be associated with clear improvements in gas exchange.

OTHER THERAPIES

EXTRACORPOREAL MEMBRANE OXYGENATION (ECMO)

ECMO is a highly specialised therapy similar to cardiopulmonary bypass for cardiac surgery. Following the H1 N1 pandemic and recent technological advances, its use is increasing. The extracorporeal circuit requires anticoagulation, usually with heparin, and is effective at both adding O_2 and removing CO_2 from the blood. The CESAR trial showed mortality benefit with transfer of patients with ARDS of less than seven days duration to a specialist centre.

EXTRACORPOREAL CO_2 REMOVAL

A drive to further decrease tidal volumes to 3.5–5 mL/kg without the side effects of hypercapnia has reopened interest in the use of an extra corporeal circuit for sole CO_2 removal. This can be undertaken with a single veno-venous catheter with an APTT of 1.5–2 times baseline. Despite sound physiological reasoning, further clinical data is needed before this becomes routine use.

OUTCOME

ARDS remains a devastating disease. Mortality has improved but still remains in excess of 30%. Outcome is dependent on the precipitant pathology. ARDS with an extrapulmonary cause (e.g. sepsis) is associated with a worse mortality than a pulmonary cause reflecting multi-organ involvement. Survivors often have some pulmonary fibrosis and reduced lung diffusing capacity resulting in some functional respiratory impairment. A significant proportion of survivors may have no impairment at all.

CLINICAL SCENARIO

In this case, the patient was transferred to intensive care where, despite recruitment manoeuvres, inverse ratio ventilation and high PEEP, she continued to require high oxygen requirements.

A decision was made to prone her within 36 hours, which led to a dramatic improvement in oxygenation. Her fluid balance was kept neutral and she was weaned from the ventilator six days after admission to intensive care. She was discharged to the respiratory ward two days after extubation. A viral throat swab was positive for influenza A.

KEY LEARNING POINTS

- Understand the definition and pathophysiology of ARDS.
- Understand how to tailor invasive ventilatory strategies to further reduce lung injury and reduce mortality.
- Understand the outcomes for patients with ARDS.

FURTHER READING

Brower, Roy G., Michael A. Matthay, Alan Morris, David Schoenfeld, B. Taylor Thompson, and Arthur Wheeler, for the Acute Respiratory Distress (ARDS) Network. "Ventilation with Lower Tidal Volumes as Compared with Traditional Tidal Volumes for Acute Lung Injury and the Acute Respiratory Distress Syndrome." *New England Journal of Medicine* 342, no. 18 (May 2000): 1301–1308.

Ferguson, Niall D., Deborah J. Cook, Gordon H. Guyatt, Sangeeta Mehta, Lori Hand, Peggy Austin, Qi Zhou, Andrea Matte, Stephen D. Walter, François Lamontagne, John T. Granton, Yaseen M. Arabi, Alejandro C. Arroliga, Thomas E. Stewart, Arthur S. Slutsky, and Maureen O. Meade, for the OSCILLATE Trial Investigators and the Canadian Critical Care Trials Group. "High-Frequency Oscillation in Early Acute Respiratory Distress Syndrome." *New England Journal of Medicine* 368, no. 9 (February 2013): 795–805.

Guérin, Claude, Jean Reignier, Jean-Christophe Richard, Pascal Beuret, Arnaud Gacouin, Thierry Boulain, Emmanuelle Mercier, Michel Badet, Alain Mercat, Olivier Baudin, Marc Clavel, Delphine Chatellier, Samir Jaber, Sylvène Rosselli, Jordi Mancebo, Michel Sirodot, Gilles Hilbert, Christian Bengler, Jack Richecoeur, Marc Gainnier, Frédérique Bayle, Gael Bourdin, Véronique Leray, Raphaele Girard, Loredana Baboi, and Louis Ayzac, for the PROSEVA Study Group. "Prone Positioning in Severe Acute Respiratory Distress Syndrome (PROSEVA)." *New England Journal of Medicine* 368, no. 23 (June 2013): 2159–2168.

41

Sepsis

DANIEL SHUTTLEWORTH AND RON DANIELS

Mr Kay is a 65-year-old man in Bed 6 who has just been admitted from the Emergency Department (ED) with a history of abdominal pain, jaundice and pyrexia of 39°C. What is your treatment plan?

This patient has presented with ascending cholangitis and has developed sepsis.

Sepsis is common in intensive care; it is a common precipitant of acute illness necessitating admission to the intensive care unit (ICU), and complicates stays.

ICU departments are characterised by some of the sickest patients, and are responsible for the highest per capita rates of antibiotic use in the hospital. Although the majority of patients develop sepsis in response to a community-acquired infection, patients in the ICU are at high risk of developing sepsis, and are more likely to be exposed to the risks associated with multi-drug resistance.

WHAT IS SEPSIS?

Sepsis can be thought of as a series of physiological responses to the presence of an infection, culminating in organ system dysfunction or failure, with potential long-term consequences among its survivors. It is not a single disease process, but a complex syndrome involving as yet ill-defined interactions between host and pathogen.

Sepsis has been defined as the presence of the systemic inflammatory response or SIRS, in the presence of a known or suspected source of infection. Severe sepsis was defined as sepsis with organ system dysfunction and septic shock, a subset of severe sepsis, where hypotension and high lactate levels persist despite adequate fluid resuscitation.

SIRS criteria (two or more of the following):

1. Temperature >38°C or <36°C
2. Heart rate >90/min
3. Respiratory rate >20/min or $PaCO_2$ <32 mmHg
4. WCC >12 or >10% immature band forms

Additional SIRS criteria were added in 2001 to include hyperglycaemia (glucose >7.7 mmol/L) in the absence of diabetes mellitus and the presence of an acutely altered mental state.

Severe sepsis criteria (sepsis plus any one of the following):

1. SBP <90 mmHg or MAP <65 mmHg or lactate >2.0 mmol/L (after initial fluid challenge)
2. INR >1.5 or a PTT >60 s
3. Bilirubin >34 μmoL/L
4. Urine output <0.5 mL/kg/hr for 2 h
5. Creatinine >177 μmoL/L
6. Platelets <100 × 10^9/L
7. SpO_2 <90% on room air

It has long been recognised that SIRS is an imperfect qualifier of sepsis. In hospital populations, many exhibit SIRS but do not develop other clinical features of sepsis. In one study, one in eight patients with infection and new organ system dysfunction criteria did not meet current criteria for diagnosis of sepsis.

In 2016, sepsis was defined by the third consensus task force as a 'life-threatening organ dysfunction due to a dysregulated host response to infection'. The 'official' definition of sepsis changed two points in the quick SOFA (Sequential Organ Failure Assessment) score in the context of infection and can be defined as

1. The presence of a known or suspected infection
2. Two or more of the following organ dysfunction criteria:
   a.   Respiratory rate >22/min
   b.   Systolic BP <100 mmHg
   c.   Altered mental status (any GCS <15)

It should be noted that subsequent validation of this assessment framework suggest that existing 'track and trigger' systems may be as or more effective in detecting the deteriorating patient.

Septic shock represents a condition of cellular and metabolic stress associated with worse outcomes when compared with the rest of the sepsis population and can be defined as

1. Persistent hypotension, with vasopressors required to support a mean arterial pressure >65 mmHg
   AND
2. Lactate >2 mmol/L, despite adequate fluid resuscitation.

HOW DO PATIENTS WITH SEPSIS PRESENT?

Patients are likely to present to the hospital with systemic manifestations of an infective process, such as pyrexia, rigors, tachycardia, tachypnoea and altered level of consciousness. They may also present with symptoms and signs relating to the site of the underlying infectious process, such as:

- Lung – Cough, dyspnoea, chest pain and sputum production
- Genitourinary tract – Dysuria, discharge, abdominal/flank pain
- Skin and soft tissue – Rashes, erythema, skin breakdown, joint pain
- Central nervous system – Headaches, convulsions, photophobia, neck pain
- GI tract – Diarrhoea, vomiting, abdominal pain, jaundice

HOW IS SEPSIS MANAGED?

Once recognised, sepsis should be considered a medical emergency. Clinical studies have shown that delays, particularly in initial resuscitation of the patient with sepsis, and in the administration of antimicrobial therapies, have been associated with dramatically worse outcomes.

Most centres use a protocolised approach to the management of sepsis incorporating input from microbiology, intensive care and admitting medical teams to optimise therapy for the local patient population and the local hospital setting. It is wise to familiarise yourself with any such protocol and use it as a starting point for your management of a patient like Mr Kay.

INITIAL RESUSCITATION

Initial resuscitation in sepsis, as with most other critically ill patients, follows a classical ABCDE approach.

- Airway
  - Ensure airway compromise is neither present nor imminent.
- Breathing
  - Assess the patient's chest; signs may be present indicating a pulmonary focus of infection.
  - Assess the amount of work the patient is doing in breathing (Respiratory rate, accessory muscle use, fatigue), and assess the efficacy of that breathing (check oxygen saturations and/or blood gases).
  - Apply oxygen if appropriate (aim for saturations of at least 94% if there is no risk of chronic CO_2 retention).
  - Consider the use of non-invasive or invasive ventilation if there is severe compromise unresponsive to basic measures.
- Circulation
  - Look for signs of vasodilation due to sepsis – a warm periphery, bounding pulses, tachycardia >90/min.
  - Look for signs of a collapsed or collapsing circulation – a cold, clammy periphery, hypotension (systolic BP <100 mmHg), weak or thready pulse, poor urine output (<0.5 mL/kg/hr) and rising serum lactate.
  - If circulatory compromise is identified, commence intravenous fluids in the form of a 250- to 500-mL bolus and assess the response. This can be repeated as necessary with suitable monitoring in place to a maximum of 30 mL/kg. Serial lactates should be measured.

- **D**isability
  - Look for the presence of depressed consciousness.
  - Also look for the presence of altered mental status. This may be less easy to spot, and clues from family, carers and nursing staff may be useful; this is often an early sign in evolving sepsis.
  - Check the patient's capillary glucose level.
- Exposure
  - Look for any potential clues to the source of sepsis; this might include open wounds, evidence of cellulitis, recent surgery, invasive procedures or trauma or presence of pain in the abdomen. Also look for indwelling catheters, cannulas and drains; all of these are potential routes for pathogens to enter.
  - Obtain cultures of blood, and where indicated urine, sputum, CSF and wound exudate.

Previous teaching suggested a rigorous early goal directed therapy (EGDT) approach to the management of septic shock, directed at rapid 'normalisation' of physiology. This approach aimed to achieve specific targets:

- Central venous pressure 8–12 mmHg (A measure of the patient's overall intravascular filling state)
- Mean arterial pressure >65 mmHg (Normalisation of vascular relaxation present in sepsis)
- Urine output of at least 0.5 mL/kg/hr
- Administration of blood products and/or inotropic therapy to achieve central venous oxygen saturations greater than 70%

Subsequent clinical studies have suggested, however, that such a rigorous goal directed approach offers little advantage over standard resuscitation. The central principles remain the correction of hypovolaemia, administration of vasopressors to correct hypotension and assessing for and correcting low cardiac output states.

Once in the ICU, patients may receive further intravenous fluids to optimise filling. This is usually continued in rapid boluses of 250–500 mL, and the effects on parameters such as CVP, mental state, urine output, lactate and peripheral temperatures observed. This process may be repeated, usually to a maximum of 30 mL/kg of fluid administered. Beyond this point, further IV fluid may become detrimental and invasive monitoring should be instituted.

A mean arterial blood pressure of 65 mmHg is sought as this represents a midpoint in the autoregulatory range of most organ system vascular beds; a higher target may be sought in hypertensive patients. The objective here is to ensure the organ systems receive an adequate supply of oxygenated blood.

Catecholamine based vasopressor drugs such as metaraminol (usually in the short term) or noradrenaline are normally used to accomplish this, with the latter requiring a central venous catheter for administration. In refractory cases, where high doses of noradrenaline fail to achieve this despite adequate filling, other drugs such as vasopressin and hydrocortisone may be added. In some cases, where cardiac function is felt to be depressed, either by sepsis directly, or by exacerbation of pre-existing cardiac disease, inotropic agents such as adrenaline or dobutamine may also be added.

ANTIMICROBIAL THERAPY

Early administration of antimicrobials is crucial in managing sepsis. Although it is desirable to obtain microbiological specimens prior to antibiotic administration, this may not always be possible and administration of antibiotics within the first hour should be the goal.

In most cases, the initial antibiotic therapy will be empirical, designed to cover most potential causative organisms and may include a beta-lactam or extended-spectrum beta-lactam, in combination with an aminoglycoside and/or nitroimidazole. Such regimens cover most Gram negatives and positives including anaerobes.

It is important to remember that antibiotics should be reviewed daily and the aim should be to rationalise agents to cover the causative organism as soon as possible, and then to discontinue treatment as soon as clinically appropriate. Excessive use of broad-spectrum antimicrobials may be harmful to the patient, by disrupting their normal microbiome and increasing the patients' vulnerability to secondary infections such as *Clostridium difficile*. Excessive broad-spectrum antibiotics also increase the selection of resistant organisms and hence pose a wider risk to society. The control of any source of infection, such as an abscess or infected indwelling catheter, is crucial in preventing unnecessary antibiotic usage.

It is extremely useful to review the patient's previous microbiological records to ascertain which antibiotics they may have been exposed to recently and whether they are known to be colonised with resistant organisms, such as MRSA. It is also important to elicit any history of allergy or intolerance.

SOME CONTROVERSIES IN SEPSIS

PARACETAMOL FOR PYREXIA IN SEPSIS

One of the questions you may be asked is 'His temperature is 38.5; can I give him some paracetamol?'

It is postulated that pyrexia may be beneficial for the immune system and detrimental to pathogens, but may also be damaging to the organ systems in the face of shock.

There are arguments each way: in the conscious patient who is uncomfortable, the analgesic properties of paracetamol are useful, as the antipyretic properties in the patient where pyrexia may be particularly damaging, such as the brain injured or post-cardiac arrest patient.

Outside these patient populations, however, there is probably little benefit gained from controlling pyrexia in sepsis in terms of mortality or length of stay in the ICU.

ACTIVATED PROTEIN C (APC)

Activated protein C (drotrecogin alfa) showed initial promise in the management of patients with severe sepsis due to its anti-inflammatory, antithrombotic and profibrinolytic properties. However, subsequent clinical trials have failed to replicate this benefit, and questions have been raised about the validity of the initial trial methodology. As a consequence, APC is no longer available in the United Kingdom.

GLYCAEMIC CONTROL

Patients with sepsis commonly develop hyperglycaemia as a consequence of disordered homeostasis in the face of excessive glucocorticoid production. It is known that uncontrolled hyperglycaemia is associated with worse outcomes, and insulin is used to maintain normoglycaemia. However, when tight glycaemic control, (aiming to maintain glucose levels at 4–7 mmol/L) is compared with less rigid regimes maintaining glucose levels at 4–11 mmol/L, the former is associated with more hypoglycaemic events and higher mortality.

WHAT ABOUT MR KAY?

Mr Kay is given antibiotics and fluids. His blood pressure drops necessitating ICU admission. He is given noradrenaline through a central line and antibiotics are continued. An ultrasound scan shows gall stones and an ERCP is performed.

Over the next three days, Mr Kay makes a good recovery and is discharged from intensive care.

KEY LEARNING POINTS

- Sepsis is a medical emergency and necessitates rapid assessment and resuscitation.
- It represents a significant amount of ICU workload.
- The best outcomes in sepsis come from normalisation of physiological variables with the objective of optimising tissue oxygen delivery, whilst minimising the complications associated with ICU treatment.

FURTHER READING

National Institute for Health and Care Excellence. *Sepsis: Recognition, Diagnosis and Early Management.* NICE Guideline NG51, National Institute for Health and Care Excellence, Manchester, UK, July 2016. www.nice.org.uk/guidance/ng51/resources/sepsis-recognition -diagnosis-and-early-management-1837508256709 (accessed 13 February 2017).

Singer, Mervyn, Clifford S. Deutschman, Christopher Warren Seymour, Manu Shankar-Hari, Djillali Annane, Michael Bauer, Rinaldo Bellomo, Gordon R. Bernard, Jean-Daniel Chiche, Craig M. Coopersmith, Richard S. Hotchkiss, Mitchell M. Levy, John C. Marshall, Greg S. Martin, Steven M. Opal, Gordon D. Rubenfeld, Tom van der Poll, Jean-Louis Vincent, and Derek C. Angus. "The Third International Consensus Definitions for Sepsis and Septic Shock (Sepsis-3)." *Journal of the American Medical Association* 315, no. 9 (February 2016): 801–810.

Young, Paul, Manoj Saxena, Rinaldo Bellomo, Ross Freebaim, Naomi Hammond, Frank van Haren, Mark Holliday, Seton Henderson, Diane Mackle, Colin McArthur, Shay McGuinness, John Myburgh, Mark Weatherall, Steve Webb, and Richard Beasley, for the HEAT Investigators and the Australian and New Zealand Intensive Care Society Clinical Trials Group. "Acetaminophen for Fever in Critically Ill Patients with Suspected Infection." *New England Journal of Medicine* 373, no. 23 (December 2015): 2215–2224.

42

Acute renal failure in intensive care (Acute kidney injury)

NITIN ARORA AND SHONDIPON K. LAHA

'Mr Jones in Bed 12 has only passed 15 mL of urine in the last three hours. What do you want us to do?'

This is one of the most common questions you are likely to be asked in intensive care on a night shift. Other specialties think we are obsessed with urine output – and they are right!

There are two main categories of renal failure: *acute* and *chronic* renal failure. We predominantly get cases of acute renal failure that occasionally evolve into the other.

Renal failure affects a number of patients in intensive care and carries significant morbidity and mortality. The prognosis is worse when renal failure occurs as part of multi-organ failure (mortality >60% if renal replacement therapy is needed).

WHAT CAUSES RENAL FAILURE?

Acute renal failure on the intensive care unit is generally multifactorial in origin. The causes can be as described in the following sections.

PRE-RENAL (GENERALLY BECAUSE OF POOR RENAL PERFUSION)

- Volume depletion
- Severe hypotension
- Reduced cardiac output
- Renovascular disease, e.g. renal artery stenosis

RENAL

- Toxaemia (sepsis, iatrogenic (drugs), rhabdomyolysis)
- Hypoxia (sepsis, ARDS, cardiogenic shock)
- Vascular (Wegener's granulomatosis, atherosclerosis)
- Pre-existing glomerulonephritis

Post-renal — obstructive causes. Rarer but we do see them

- Blocked urinary catheter
- Enlarged prostate
- Increased abdominal pressure (compartment syndrome)
- Malignancy

DIAGNOSIS OF ACUTE RENAL FAILURE/ACUTE KIDNEY INJURY (AKI)

Diagnosed on the basis of history and biochemical investigations. There should be

- Abrupt onset (less than 48 hours).
- Deterioration of kidney function characterised by rise in serum creatinine (>50% from baseline or increase by 25 mmol/L) and oliguria (<0.5 mL/kg/hr for more than six hours).

Staging

Different systems of staging acute kidney injury (AKI) are available. They include the AKIN (Acute Kidney Injury Network), RIFLE and Kidney Disease Improving Global Outcomes (KDIGO) criteria. All of these criteria are mainly based on a rise in creatinine and urine output. The most commonly used in our ICUs is *RIFLE* (Risk, Injury, Failure, Loss, End stage renal disease):

R(isk) of AKI – Rise in serum creatinine by >50% from baseline or urine output <0.5 mL/kg/hr for six hours

I(njury) – Rise in serum creatinine by >100% from baseline or urine output <0.5 mL/kg/hr for more than 12 hours

F(ailure) – Rise in serum creatinine by 300% from baseline or increase by >350 μmol/L; or urine output <0.3 mL/kg/hr for 24 hours or anuria for 12 hours

L(oss) – Persistent loss of kidney function for four weeks
E(nd stage renal disease) – Loss of kidney function for more than three
months

If two criteria do not match the same stage of severity, the worse one is used.

HOW DO I PREVENT RENAL FAILURE?

There is no easy answer. First identify the risk factors. Sometimes we can modulate the body's response on the ICU with fluid optimisation and other interventions or by more frequent monitoring of risks (e.g. intra-abdominal pressure). Occasionally renal failure may be inevitable and early planning of management will avoid worsening this.

INVESTIGATIONS

BLOODS

- *Urea and Creatinine*
  Definitive levels that indicate renal failure are very unreliable but an increasing trend in both is highly suggestive. If the ratio of urea to creatinine rises, this suggests a pre-renal cause.
- *Potassium*
  Acute renal failure can often cause raised potassium levels (which may also be reflected on the ECG).
- *Haemoglobin*
  An increase in haemoglobin and haematocrit suggests very concentrated blood and dehydration.
- *Blood gases*
  Increasing negative base excess, acidosis and rising lactate are all suggestive of possible renal failure causing metabolic acidosis.
- *Creatinine Clearance*
  Creatinine is an inert substance predominantly filtered by the glomerulus. It has a relatively constant plasma rate and is routinely measured. Its clearance allows an approximation of glomerular filtration rate but may

be approximately 10% above actual GFR (due to not recognising the component of secreted creatinine).

This is normally over a 24-hour period but many units will do this over six hours providing a quicker but less accurate result.

URINE

- Proteins, blood, urine sodium, osmolality, microscopy and culture

OTHER INVESTIGATIONS

Other investigations including radiography should be guided by clinical suspicion of cause.

WHAT DO YOU DO IN RESPONSE TO THE NURSE'S QUESTION? (TREATMENT OF ACUTE RENAL FAILURE)

INITIAL TREATMENT (WITHIN SIX HOURS)

REMEMBER YOUR ABC

1. Make sure the airway is patent.
2. Give 100% oxygen until the patient is in a stable environment and his respiratory history can be assessed.
3. Make sure there is adequate large bore venous access. Does the patient look clinically hypovolaemic? If so, give a bolus of fluid (Crystalloid or colloid).
4. Treat hyperkalaemia with calcium gluconate or an insulin/dextrose regime (there is normally a hospital protocol for this).

LINES

Often these patients will need a central venous catheter for assessing fluid status and for vasopressor support if required. An arterial line may be required. These patients should have a urinary catheter in situ with hourly urine outputs being measured.

DRUGS

- *Diuretics* (Furosemide): Occasionally used once the patient is well filled to induce diuresis (but be wary as this may cause further renal damage).
- *Sodium Bicarbonate*: This is occasionally used as a temporary holding measure to correct a metabolic acidosis. Do not use it without senior advice.
- Stop or minimise nephrotoxic drugs if possible.

RENAL REPLACEMENT THERAPY

Renal replacement therapy (RRT) is the treatment of established renal failure that has not responded to the above initial measures. Major indications for renal replacement therapy are

- Fluid overload leading to pulmonary oedema not responding to diuretics
- Hyperkalaemia unresponsive to medical management
- Severe metabolic acidosis
- Oliguria or anuria
- Rising urea and creatinine
- Drug overdose with a substance amenable to removal by dialysis

Renal replacement therapy seeks to artificially mimic the excretory function of the kidney. The common thread among all methods is use of a semipermeable membrane for filtration.

Various modes of delivering renal replacement therapy include

- Peritoneal dialysis
- Haemodialysis
- Haemofiltration

For a more detailed explanation of renal replacement therapy, refer to Chapter 24.

CONCOMITANT MEDICATION

Drug pharmacokinetics in patients on renal replacement therapy can be very complex and differ from patients not on renal replacement. Dose and frequency of administration also vary between haemodialysis and haemofiltration. If in doubt, expert advice must be sought from the renal physicians, renal drug handbook or a renal pharmacist.

LONG-TERM PROGNOSIS

Nearly two-thirds of acute renal failure patients that survive to discharge will regain most of their renal function. However, about 15%–30% need continuing renal replacement therapy after discharge from the unit so they must be referred to, and managed jointly with renal physicians.

KEY LEARNING POINTS

- Causes of acute renal failure can be classified into pre-renal, post-renal and renal groups.
- Diagnosis is based on history, clinical examination and changes in biochemistry.
- AKI can be staged using *RIFLE*.
- Treatment is split into initial management and renal replacement therapy.

FURTHER READING

Acute Dialysis Quality Initiative website. www.adqi.org/Home-Call.htm

Intensive Care Society. "Standards and Recommendations for the Provision of Renal Replacement Therapy on Intensive Care Units in the United Kingdom." Guideline. Intensive Care Society, London, UK, January 2009.

Kellum, John A., Rinaldo Bellomo, and Claudio Ronco. "Definition and Classification of Acute Kidney Injury." *Nephron Clinical Practice* 109, no. 4 (September 2008): c182–c187.

National Institute for Health and Care Excellence (NICE). "Acute Kidney Injury: Prevention, Detection and Management up to the Point of Renal Replacement Therapy." Clinical guideline CG169, National Institute for Health and Care Excellence, Manchester, UK, August 2013. www.nice.org.uk/guidance/cg169/evidence/acute-kidney-injury-full -guideline-191530621 (accessed 1 September 2016).

Ronco, Claudio, Rinaldo Bellomo, Peter Homel, Alessandra Brendolan, Maurizio Dan, Pasquale Piccinni, and Giuseppe La Greca. "Effects of Different Doses in Continuous Veno-Venous Haemofiltration on Outcomes of Acute Renal Failure: A Prospective Randomised Trial." *Lancet* 355 (July 2000): 26–30.

43

Management of severe acute pancreatitis

LAURA DYAL AND FANG GAO

You are the SHO asked to review 60-year-old Mr Graham. He presented two days ago with epigastric pain and vomiting. He has a history of alcohol excess. He was diagnosed with acute pancreatitis and started on pain relief and IV fluids. Forty-eight hours later, the nursing staff are concerned as he looks much more unwell, and is hypotensive and oliguric.

Why might this patient require intensive care support and what treatment can be offered?

Acute pancreatitis is an inflammatory disorder of the pancreas where pancreatic enzymes leak out from the acinar cells to surrounding pancreatic tissues and cause an acute inflammatory response (Young and Thompson, 2008).

The condition can be viewed as a four-stage process and resolution can occur at any point in the sequence of events (Charnley, 2005).

1. Oedema and fluid shifts, which can lead to hypovolaemic shock.
2. Fluids and enzymes leak into peritoneal cavity and can cause auto digestion of fats – leading to fat necrosis.
3. Autodigestion can affect the blood vessels – this can cause bleeding and is responsible for the bruising as blood tracks along the retroperitoneal space – e.g. bruising in the flanks (Grey–Turner's sign) and at the umbilicus (Cullen's sign).
4. Inflammation can lead to necrosis. The infected necrosis is associated with a higher mortality rate (Charnley, 2005).

Around 80% of acute pancreatitis is mild, self-limiting and resolves with simple supportive management. Severe acute pancreatitis (SAP) accounts for 20% of cases and is associated with organ dysfunction. Hospital mortality in patients with infected pancreatic necrosis is threefold higher than without infected necrosis (Banks and Freeman, 2006).

SYMPTOMS/SIGNS

- Severe constant epigastric pain – radiating to back/flanks
- Vomiting
- Pyrexia
- Abdominal distension
- Grey–Turner's/Cullen's sign – not always seen
- Signs of end organ involvement
  - Oliguria
  - Jaundice
  - Respiratory distress

CAUSES

Acronym to remember the causes of pancreatitis:

- **I** – Idiopathic
- **G** – Gallstone
- **E** – Ethanol
- **T** – Trauma
- **S** – Steroids
- **M** – Malignancy, mumps and other viral infections (Coxsackie B, Epstein–Barr, mycoplasma, HIV-related co-infections)
- **A** – Autoimmune – e.g. systemic lupus erythematosus (SLE)
- **S** – Scorpion bites
- **H** – Hyperlipidaemia (hyperparathyroidism, hypercalcaemia, hypothermia, hereditary conditions)
- **E** – Endoscopic retrograde cholangiopancreatography (ERCP; 2–3% of cases)
- **D** – Drugs – e.g. furosemide, azathioprine, thiazide diuretics

INVESTIGATIONS

Test	Result
Serum lipase	Elevated (more sensitive and specific than amylase) – levels start to peak 4–8 hours after pain and remain for 8–14 days
Serum amylase	Three times the upper limit of normal – raised 2–12 hours after onset of pain with peak at 48 hours and returns to normal 3–5 days after pain started
AST/ALT	If >3x, normal increased likelihood of gallstones pancreatitis
Full blood count	Raised white cell count (WCC)
Arterial blood gas	Hypoxaemia and acid–base disturbance
Abdominal X-ray	May see sentinel loop – adjacent to the pancreas – as the bowel near the pancreas becomes oedematous
Chest X-ray	Atelectasis/pleural effusion (especially left side)
Ultrasound	Pancreatic inflammation, peripancreatic stranding, fluid collections
C-reactive protein	The higher, the more likely pancreatic necrosis

Test	Result
Abdominal CT	Irregularity of pancreas, obliteration of peripancreatic fat, necrosis/pseudocysts
MRCP	Gallstones, pseudocysts, obliteration of perinephric fat
ERCP	Identification/removal of gallstones – however, cause for pancreatitis in 2%–3% of ERCPs performed
Fine needle aspiration	To identify causative organism in infected pancreatitis
Urinary trypsinogen	New marker – this is 94% sensitive with 95% specificity and now considered a better screening test than amylase

Source: Daley et al., 2015.

SCORING SYSTEMS

How severe is the pancreatitis? Is your patient at risk of death?

There are scoring systems available to describe severity of acute pancreatitis or to predict mortality. They are not used for diagnosis.

The scores are derived from the clinical picture, biochemical investigations and also radiological imaging.

RANSON'S CRITERIA

Severity criteria are divided into gallstone and non-gallstone pancreatitis (Ranson et al., 1976).

NON-GALLSTONE PANCREATITIS

Criteria on hospital admission	Score
Age > 55 y	1
Glucose > 11.1 mmol	1
WCC > **16 (× 10⁹/L)**	1
Serum AST > 250 units/L	1
Serum LDH > 350 units/L	1

Criteria after 48 hours since admission	Score
HCT fall > 10%	1
Estimated fluid sequestration > 6 L	1

Criteria after 48 hours since admission	Score
Base deficit > 4 mEq/L	1
Blood urea nitrogen rise > 1.8 mmol/L	1
Serum calcium < 2 mmol	1
PO_2 < 8 kPa	1

GALLSTONE PANCREATITIS

Differences highlighted in bold.

Criteria on admission	Score
Age > 70 y	1
Glucose **> 12.2 mmol/L**	1
WCC **> 18 (× 10⁹/L)**	1
Serum AST > 250 units/L	1
Serum LDH **> 400 units/L**	1

Criteria after 48 hours	Score
HCT fall >10%	1
Estimated fluid sequestration **> 4 L**	1
Blood urea nitrogen rise **> 0.7 mmol/L**	1
Serum calcium < 2 mmol/L	1

Ranson's scores and related mortality (%) for both gallstone and non-gallstone pancreatitis are approximated as

- *0–2 = 0%*
- *3–4 = 15%*
- *5–6 = 50%*
- *> 6 = 100%*

'GLASCOW' CRITERIA

G – Glucose > 10 mmol
L – LDH > 600 units/L
A – Age > 55 years
S – Serum albumin < 32 g/L and serum urea
        Serum urea nitrogen > 16.1 mmol/L

C – Calcium < 2 mmol/L

O – Oxygen pressure (arterial) < 8 kPa in air

W – WCC > 15

A point for each parameter.

Score < 2 = Mild acute pancreatitis

Score = 2 = Moderate acute pancreatitis

Score > 3 = Severe acute pancreatitis

BACK TO THE PATIENT

Mr Graham has heart rate of 140 beats per minute, BP of 90/50 mmHg, and looks pale and clammy. His urine output has been poor despite several litres of fluid resuscitation. He is working hard to breathe and his ABG shows hypoxia and acidosis.

Q1: What would you do now?

Mr Graham is showing signs of end organ dysfunction. He is likely to be developing severe acute pancreatitis. His clinical condition must be discussed with seniors and an intensive care doctor should review him to consider offering him supportive treatment.

Q2: What are the strong indicators for critical care admission in a patient with severe acute pancreatitis?

Strong indications for admission to a critical care unit with those fulfilling the diagnosis of severe acute pancreatitis include

1. Ongoing need for fluid resuscitation
2. Age > 70 years
3. BMI > 30
4. Presence of indicators of more severe disease
   a. Necrosis of > 30% of pancreas
   b. Pleural effusions
   c. Three or more of Ranson's criteria present
   d. CRP > 150 at 48 hours (Nathens et al., 2004)

Q3: What is the management of severe acute pancreatitis in the intensive care unit?

The treatment is supportive. Patients with severe acute pancreatitis may need a number of organ systems to be supported.

RESPIRATORY

Inflammation of the pancreas can cause diaphragmatic splinting, pleural effusions and acute lung injury. Patients will become hypoxic, often develop respiratory failure and require invasive respiratory support with intubation and ventilation.

CARDIOVASCULAR

Despite fluid resuscitation, patients can still be depleted due to increased losses, and leaky capillary membranes. Careful fluid management guided using intensive haemodynamic monitoring is a reason to admit to intensive care unit. Central access may be required and cardiac output monitoring can be used to help guide fluid replacement. Patients may also require cardiovascular support with vasopressors such as noradrenaline, especially if peripherally dilated and septic.

RENAL

Renal failure is common and hourly monitoring of urine output is essential. Patients need an adequate perfusion pressure to ensure adequate blood flow to the kidneys and other organs. If renal failure does develop, haemofiltration may be required.

NUTRITION

Meeting the metabolic demands and nutritional needs is paramount. Early enteral feeding – ideally gastric is required. If gastric feeding is not tolerated due pancreatic gastric irritation or pancreatic mass causing obstruction, Nasojejunal (NJ) feeding may be required. Some patients may need parenteral nutrition. If the cause of pancreatitis is alcohol, ensure vitamins such as thiamine are given.

MANAGEMENT OF PSEUDOCYSTS AND INFECTION

Pseudocysts are encapsulated collections of pancreatic fluid. They can become infected or rupture and some can cause haemorrhage. The treatment options include the preferred conservative management but if the cyst becomes infected, surgical options include excision of cyst, external drainage or internal drainage with Roux-en-Y cystojejunostomy, cystogastrostomy, or cystoduodenostomy.

Antibiotics are only indicated if sepsis is suspected or if blood cultures or drain fluid cultures show bacterial growth. Routine antibiotic prophylaxis is not indicated. Bacterial infection (mostly *E. coli*) is the cause of up to 80% of deaths in the severe acute pancreatitis group. The antibiotics of choice are carbapenems, which have good broad-spectrum coverage.

SURGICAL MANAGEMENT

Early surgical intervention in severe acute pancreatitis has a very high mortality. The surgical team aims to manage the patient with full supportive therapy on ICU and try all other methods of improving the patient's condition before resorting to surgical intervention (Young and Thompson, 2008). Surgery in pancreatitis is only used to

1. Relieve biliary obstruction
2. Minimise the damage to other organs
3. Remove infected intra- and extrahepatic necrosis

KEY LEARNING POINTS

- Acute pancreatitis can be a life-threatening condition.
- Treatment is generally supportive but surgery may be needed for some patients.
- Nutrition must be addressed. Most patients will tolerate enteral nutrition but some may need parenteral nutrition.

FURTHER READING

Banks, Peter A., and Martin L. Freeman, for the Practice Parameters Committee of the American College of Gastroenterology. "Practice Guidelines in Acute Pancreatitis." *American Journal of Gastroenterology* 101 (2006): 2379–2400.

Charnley, Richard M. "Liver, Biliary Tract and Pancreas." In *Surgical Talk*. 2nd ed., edited by Andrew Goldberg and Gerard Stansby, 79–104. London: Imperial College Press; 2005.

Daley, Brian, Catherine L. McKnight, and Jose F. Aycinena. "Acute Pancreatitis." *BMJ Best Practice*. London: BMJ Publishing Group. 2015.

Nathens, Avery B., J. Randall Curtis; Richard J. Beale; Deborah J. Cook; Rui P. Moreno; Jacques-André Romand; Shawn J. Skerrett; Renee D. Stapleton; Lorraine B. Ware; and Carl S. Waldmann. "Management of the Critically Ill Patient with Severe Acute Pancreatitis." *Critical Care Medicine* 32, no. 12 (December 2004): 2524–2536.

Ranson, John H., Kenneth M. Rifkind, and James W. Turner. "Prognostic Signs and Nonoperative Peritoneal Lavage in Acute Pancreatitis." *Surgery, Gynecology & Obstetrics* 143, no. 2 (1976): 209–219.

Young, Simon P., and Jonathan P. Thompson. "Severe Acute Pancreatitis." *Continuing Education in Anaesthesia, Critical Care & Pain* 8, no. 4 (2008): 125–128.

Hepatic failure

FAYAZ BABA AND MARK PUGH

You are called to the emergency department to see a 45-year-old male with a history of taking 20 tablets of paracetamol. Four hours have passed and now the patient has nausea and vomiting.

What things are going through your mind?
What complications are you expecting and how you are going to deal with this patient?
This chapter aims to help you answer these questions.

Acute liver failure is a rare but life-threatening critical illness in which there is rapid deterioration of liver function in a previously healthy individual. The involvement of other organs makes acute liver failure an extremely difficult condition to manage. The intensive care unit (ICU) has a pivotal role in the management of this condition by providing support for failing organs while allowing time for hepatic regeneration or for pre-optimization prior to liver transplantation. Unfortunately, acute decompensation on the background of chronic liver disease is all too common (most commonly secondary to alcohol and, increasingly, Hepatitis C). This chapter will address normal liver function, causes of acute liver failure, how to evaluate liver function clinically and biochemically, and subsequent management and prognosis.

PHYSIOLOGY OF LIVER

The liver is the largest organ in the body and is involved in many important functions of it.

The following are the liver's major functions:

- Metabolism of fat, protein (synthesis, deamination to urea) and carbohydrate (glucose synthesis, storage in the form of glycogen and glucose production from other substrates – gluconeogenesis)

- Production and breakdown of hormones
- Removal of toxins and conversion into less harmful metabolites (including drug metabolism)
- Breakdown of red blood cells (production of bile)
- Synthesis of plasma proteins, albumin, clotting factors
- Immune function, removal of bacteria and antigens
- Storage of vitamins (A, D, B12) and essential minerals (iron and copper)

CAUSES OF LIVER FAILURE

There are numerous causes for acute hepatic failure but Paracetamol poisoning remains the leading cause in the United Kingdom.

DRUG-RELATED HEPATOTOXICITY

- Paracetamol
- Antibiotics (amoxicillin-clavulanate, ciprofloxacin, doxycycline, erythromycin, isoniazid, nitrofurantoin, tetracycline)
- Antidepressants (amitriptyline, nortriptyline)
- Antiepileptics (phenytoin, valproate)
- Anaesthetic agents (halothane)
- Lipid-lowering medications (atorvastatin, lovastatin, simvastatin)
- Immunosuppressive agents (cyclophosphamide, methotrexate)
- Nonsteroidal anti-inflammatory agents (NSAIDs)
- Salicylates (ingestion of these agents may result in Reye syndrome)

HEPATIC FAILURE IN PREGNANCY

- Acute fatty liver of pregnancy frequently culminates in fulminant hepatic failure.
- The HELLP (haemolysis, elevated liver enzymes, low platelets) syndrome occurs in 0.1%–0.6% of pregnancies. It is usually associated with preeclampsia and may rarely result in liver failure.

TOXIN-RELATED HEPATOTOXICITY

- *Amanita phalloides* mushroom toxin
- *Bacillus cereus* toxin

- Cyanobacteria toxin
- Organic solvents (e.g. carbon tetrachloride)
- Yellow phosphorus

VASCULAR CAUSES

- Ischemic hepatitis
- Hepatic vein thrombosis (Budd–Chiari syndrome)
- Hepatic veno-occlusive disease
- Portal vein thrombosis
- Hepatic arterial thrombosis (consider post transplant)

METABOLIC CAUSES

- Alpha-1antitrypsin deficiency
- Fructose intolerance
- Galactosaemia
- Lecithin-cholesterol acyltransferase deficiency
- Reye syndrome
- Wilson's disease

MALIGNANCIES

- Primary liver tumour (usually hepatocellular carcinoma, rarely cholangiocarcinoma)
- Secondary tumour (extensive hepatic metastases or lymphoma; leukaemia)

Miscellaneous causes of hepatic failure include adult-onset Still's disease, heatstroke, and primary graft non-function in liver transplant recipients.

PRESENTATION

HISTORY

History is valuable for suggesting the likely causes of acute liver failure and guiding appropriate interventions.

- Date of onset of jaundice and encephalopathy
- Medication and alcohol use

- Herbal or traditional medicine use
- Family history of liver disease (Wilson's disease)
- Exposure to risk factors for viral hepatitis
- Exposure to hepatic toxins
- Evidence of complications, e.g. renal failure, seizures, etc.

PHYSICAL EXAMINATION

Careful assessment and documentation of the patient's mental status:

- Stigmata of chronic liver disease.
- Jaundice (not always present).
- Right upper quadrant tenderness is variably present.
- The liver may be small if significant necrosis or it may be enlarged.
- Cerebral oedema may ultimately give rise to manifestations of increased intracranial pressure (ICP), including papilledema, hypertension and bradycardia.
- Rapid development of ascites, especially if observed in a patient with fulminant hepatic failure accompanied by abdominal pain, suggests the possibility of hepatic vein thrombosis (Budd–Chiari syndrome).
- Haematemesis or melaena.
- Patients can be hypotensive and tachycardic as a result of the reduced systemic vascular resistance that accompanies fulminant hepatic failure, a pattern that is indistinguishable from septic shock.
- Assessment of hepatic encephalopathy.
    - Grade I – Altered mood, euphoria or anxiety, shortened attention span
    - Grade II – Drowsy, inappropriate behaviour, minimal disorientation of time or place
    - Grade III – Somnolence, confusion, gross disorientation
    - Grade IV – Coma with or without response to painful stimuli

COMPLICATIONS

Potential complications of acute liver failure include seizures, haemorrhage, infection, renal failure and metabolic imbalances.

MANAGEMENT

The most important step in patients with acute liver failure is to identify the cause.

Prognosis in acute liver failure is dependent on aetiology.

All patients with clinical or laboratory evidence of moderate or severe acute hepatitis should have immediate measurement of prothrombin time (PT) and careful evaluation of mental status.

PROTHROMBIN TIME

The PT and/or the international normalised ratio (INR) are used to determine the presence and severity of coagulopathy. These are sensitive markers of hepatic synthetic failure.

HEPATIC ENZYMES

The levels of the hepatic enzymes are often elevated dramatically as a result of severe hepatocellular necrosis.

In instances of paracetamol toxicity (especially alcohol-enhanced), the AST and ALT level may be well over 10,000 U/L. The alkaline phosphatase (ALP) level may be normal or elevated.

SERUM BILIRUBIN

A serum bilirubin that is elevated to greater than 4 mg/dL (68 μmol/L) suggests a poor prognosis in the setting of acetaminophen poisoning.

SERUM AMMONIA

The serum ammonia level may be elevated dramatically in patients with fulminant hepatic failure.

SERUM GLUCOSE

Serum glucose levels may be dangerously low. This decrease is the result of impairments in glycogen production and gluconeogenesis.

SERUM LACTATE

Arterial blood lactate levels, either at four hours (> 3.5 mmol/L) or at twelve hours (> 3.0 mmol/L) are early predictors of outcome in paracetamol-induced acute liver failure.

OTHER USEFUL TESTS

Full blood count (FBC) may reveal thrombocytopenia
Liver ultrasonography (USG) or CT scan
Screen for hepatitis A/B/C/E
Paracetamol levels
Hepatitis screen

DIAGNOSIS

The diagnosis of acute liver failure is made with reference to the specific criteria listed below. However, the clinical picture is dominated by coagulopathy and encephalopathy.

1. Absence of chronic liver disease
2. Acute hepatitis (elevation in AST/ALT) accompanied by elevation in INR > 1.5
3. Any degree of mental alteration (encephalopathy)
4. Illness less than 26 weeks duration

MANAGEMENT OF ACUTE LIVER FAILURE

Good intensive care support is paramount in the management of acute liver failure. Patients with grade II encephalopathy should be transferred to the ICU for monitoring and generally grade III encephalopathy warrants intubation for airway protection.

MANAGEMENT OF ENCEPHALOPATHY AND CEREBRAL OEDEMA

Intubate and ventilate if risk of aspiration.

ICP monitoring (controversial) if grade III or IV encephalopathy. ICP monitoring helps in the early recognition of cerebral oedema.

Elevate head to 30 degrees to improve cerebral perfusion pressure (CPP).

The patient should be appropriately sedated to prevent stimuli from rising ICP.

Avoid hypotension. This may require use of vasoactive drugs.

Prevent hypoxaemia • Target $PaCO_2$ of 4.7–5.2 kPa (low normal range).

Tight glycaemic control with blood glucose target between 4 and 10 mmol/L.

Mannitol (0.25–0.5 g/kg) is used to treat intracranial hypertension associated with cerebral oedema.

Hypertonic saline can be utilised with similar benefits.

INFECTION

Patients are prone to get both bacterial and fungal infections. The normal systemic features of infection may be absent in patients with ALF and therefore extra vigilance is required, and if suspected, then should be treated aggressively after advice from a microbiologist.

COAGULATION

Clinically significant bleeding is not common. So monitor synthetic functions (INR) and thrombocytopenia, but generally correction is discouraged, as PT/INR are prognostic. The exception is when an invasive procedure is planned or in the presence of profound coagulopathy (INR > 7).

N-ACETYLCYSTEINE

N-acetylcysteine is used in paracetamol poisoning with proven efficacy and should be administered as soon as possible following the overdose as guided by treatment nomograms. It is widely accepted that N-acetylcysteine should be administered in all cases of ALF although the efficacy is not known.

LIVER TRANSPLANTATION

Liver transplantation is the definitive treatment in liver failure, but a detailed discussion is beyond the scope of this book.

In all cases of severe acute liver failure that do not respond to above management, seek advice from a regional liver unit. The patient may be suitable for liver transplant. The King's College Hospital criteria is probably the most widely used with the highest diagnostic accuracy (beyond the scope of this book).

DIET

If the patient is not eating and enteral feeding is not feasible (e.g. in paralytic ileus), then consider total parenteral nutrition (TPN).

Monitor blood glucose level carefully as the patient may require large amounts of IV glucose. Restricting protein to 0.6 g/kg of body weight per day was previously routine in the setting of hepatic encephalopathy. However, this may not be necessary and advice from the gastroenterologist should be sought.

PROGNOSIS

Patients meeting the criteria for liver transplantation with acute liver failure have above 80% mortality without transplantation. With transplantation, five-year survival rates are in excess of 70% and continue to improve.

Patients with acute decompensation of alcoholic liver disease have an overall poor prognosis – this raises ethical issues with regard to their admission to Critical Care, particularly if they have had an episode of decompensation previously and continue to drink despite advice to do otherwise.

CLINICAL SCENARIO – CONTINUED

Coming back to the above scenario, when called to the ED to see this patient, management will be

- ABCD approach.
- Assessment of encephalopathy and GCS may need immediate intubation.
- History and duration from ingestion.
- Differentials.
- Bloods for FBC, U&E, liver function tests including INR and prothrombin time.
- Do not correct INR unless needed. Before correcting, discuss with a senior.
- Paracetamol and salicylate levels.

- NAC according to nomogram.
- ICU/HDU support.
- Discussion with a senior and a gastroenterologist.
- If fulminant liver failure, discuss with regional liver unit. It may be appropriate for emergency liver transplant.

KEY LEARNING POINTS

- Acute liver failure is relatively uncommon.
- Liver transplant is the definitive treatment.
- Early recognition, appropriate resuscitation and early referral to a regional liver unit improve survival.

FURTHER READING

Jalan, Rajiv, Pere Gines, Jody C. Olson, Rajeshwar P. Mookerjee, Richard Moreau, Guadalupe Garcia-Tsao, Vicente Arroyo, and Patrick S. Kamath. "Acute-On Chronic Liver Failure." *Journal of Hepatology* 57 (December 2012):1336–1348.

Sood, Gagan K, Steven A. Conrad, Lemi Luu, and Mark S. Slabinski. "Acute Liver Failure." *Medscape* (updated: 4 February 2016).

Trotter, James F. "Practical Management of Acute Liver Failure in the Intensive Care Unit." *Current Opinion in Critical Care* 15, no. 2 (April 2009): 163–167.

45

Non-traumatic brain injuries

RICHARD YARDLEY AND SHASHIKUMAR CHANDRASHEKARAIAH

'Mrs Smith, the 60-year-old lady with a grade I subarachnoid haemorrhage has just arrived from the Emergency Department and her GCS has dropped. What would you like us to do?'

Unless you are working in a neurosciences centre, you will not be exposed to such patients on a regular basis. However, these patients will initially present to peripheral hospitals and need to be assessed, stabilised and transferred to a place of definitive care. Fifty to sixty per cent of patients will die in the first six months following a subarachnoid haemorrhage, and of those who survive, approximately one-third will have severe disability with lasting effects on the personal, social and financial aspects of their lives and of those around them. Although we cannot reverse the immediate damage inflicted at the time of the haemorrhage, good 'basic' critical care management and early recognition and treatment of subsequent complications will optimise the chance of a good neurological outcome.

WHAT IS A SUBARACHNOID HAEMORRHAGE AND WHAT CAUSES IT?

The arachnoid mater is the middle of the three meninges that surround the brain and spinal cord. It is attached to the dura (the outermost layer), but is separated from the innermost pia mater by the subarachnoid space, which contains cerebrospinal fluid (CSF). A subarachnoid haemorrhage (SAH) is defined as bleeding into this subarachnoid space.

SAH is classified into traumatic or non-traumatic. Causes of non-traumatic SAH are

- Rupture of intracranial aneurysm, accounting for 85% of spontaneous bleeds.
- Ten per cent of cases are non-aneurysmal and no cause is found.
- Around 5% are due to uncommon conditions such as arteriovenous malformations, tumour, coagulopathy and drug misuse.

Non-traumatic SAH has an incidence of approximately 9 cases per 100,000 population per year worldwide. It is twice as common in females, and most commonly affects the 50–65 age range. Six-month mortality is in the region of 60%. Risk factors include

- Smoking (most important risk factor, risk ratio of current smoking = 2.2).
- Alcohol excess.
- Systemic hypertension.
- Family history.
- Hereditary diseases (polycystic kidneys, connective tissue disorders).
- Anticoagulants and antiplatelet therapy probably do not increase the incidence of aneurysmal rupture, but increase the severity when it does occur.

DIAGNOSIS OF SAH

Clinical suspicion from the history, including *collateral history*, should guide subsequent focussed examination and appropriate investigations:

- Patients present with a variety of signs and symptoms, ranging from mild headache to sudden collapse and death.
- Classically there is sudden onset of a very severe occipital headache, described as 'like being hit over the head with a cricket bat'.
- Nausea and vomiting, photophobia and visual disturbance are common.
- Fifty per cent of patients will develop confusion, reduced levels of consciousness or focal neurology, and 10% will develop seizures.
- Signs often include systemic hypertension and tachycardia.
- Assess for neck stiffness (a sign of meningeal irritation) and examine the cranial nerves.
- A non-contrast CT scan is the most appropriate initial investigation as it is performed quickly and will positively identify most cases of SAH.
- A strong clinical suspicion with negative CT findings should be followed up with a lumbar puncture. Xanthochromia supports the diagnosis, though is not specific (yellow-stained CSF caused by bilirubin, a breakdown product of red blood cells, which is undetectable until 6–12 hours after the headache).
- Once the diagnosis has been made, the search for a treatable cause – usually a cerebral artery aneurysm – begins. This may involve CT, MR or digital subtraction angiography.

CLASSIFICATION OF SAH

The most important determinant of outcome following SAH is the neurological condition at *the time of admission*. The World Federation of Neurological Surgeons classifies patients with SAH according to the Glasgow Coma Scale (GCS) and the presence or absence of focal motor neurological deficit:

GCS score	Focal neurological deficit	Grade	Proportion of patients with poor outcome
15	No	1	14.8%
13–14	No	2	29.4%
13–14	Yes	3	52.6%
7–12	Yes/no	4	58.3%
3–6	Yes/no	5	92.7%

The neurological function may deteriorate due to complications *after* admission. This does not change the grade of the SAH, which is determined *at the time of admission*. Poor outcomes are seen in approximately 15% of grade 1 SAH, rising to almost 93% in grade 5.

Other determinants of poor outcome include

- Age: mortality following SAH in octogenarians is triple that in younger people
- Severity of initial bleeding
- Aneurysm site and size
- History of chronic hypertension
- High systolic blood pressure on admission
- Heavy alcohol consumption

COMPLICATIONS

DISEASE-ASSOCIATED EVENTS

- Aspiration – vomiting is common in SAH, and may be accompanied by loss of airway-protective reflexes in the neurologically obtunded patient.

- Cardiopulmonary complications – due to very high levels of circulating catecholamines following initial event. Severe hypertension, ECG changes, dysrhythmias, myocardial infarction, cardiac arrest or pulmonary oedema may occur.
- Stress hyperglycaemia – also caused by the 'catecholamine storm' and associated with poor outcomes.
- Pyrexia – without evidence of infection in 20% of cases. Attributed to inflammation around extravasated blood in the subarachnoid space. Independent risk factor for poor outcome.
- Hypercoagulability.
- Seizures.
- Hydrocephalus: dilated ventricles caused by obstruction in the flow of CSF due to location of the SAH or extension of the bleed into the ventricles themselves. Patients may exhibit poor neurological status initially.
- Delayed ischaemic deficit: due to cerebral vasospasm, which peaks around one week after the initial bleed.
- Rebleeding: If a ruptured aneurysm is left untreated, approximately one-third of patients who recover from the initial haemorrhage will die due to recurrent bleeding. Fifty per cent of recurrent bleeds will occur in the first six months.

TREATMENT-ASSOCIATED EVENTS

- Neurointervention-related complications such as air embolism, dissection and ischaemic stroke

COMPLICATIONS ASSOCIATED WITH PROLONGED BED REST

- Venous thromboembolic disease, healthcare-associated infection

MANAGEMENT

Management consists of good 'basic' critical care and appropriate, timely neurosurgical and/or neuroradiological intervention.

CRITICAL CARE

- Admission to critical care for continuous monitoring and control of airway, breathing, circulation and neurological function.
- Blood pressure: stop any antihypertensives. Although strong evidence is lacking, reducing systolic BP to below 180 mmHg until the aneurysm is treated seems sensible. Maintaining a MAP >90 mmHg is also advised.
- Avoidance of raised intracranial pressure: bed rest, analgesia, consideration of anti-emetics and laxatives.
- Seizure management: there is no evidence for prophylactic anticonvulsant therapy, but clinically apparent seizures should be treated.
- Delayed ischaemic deficit: nimodipine (a calcium antagonist) 60 mg four-hourly for three weeks is used prophylactically to reduce the occurrence of secondary ischaemia and improve neurological outcomes.
- Management of hyperglycaemia: treatment of blood glucose of more than 10 mmol/L is advised.
- Management of pyrexia: pharmacological and physical. No demonstrated benefit of inducing hypothermia.
- VTE prophylaxis: low-molecular weight heparins increase the risk of rebleeding and, therefore, pneumatic devices +/– graduated compression stockings should be employed.
- There is no robust evidence to support induced hypervolaemia and hypertension, although in practice this approach is often employed.

NEUROSURGICAL AND NEURORADIOLOGICAL INTERVENTION

- CT angiogram of the cerebral vessels to identify the ruptured vessel and plan appropriate intervention.
- Primary goal of treatment is occlusion of the ruptured aneurysm.
- Two options available: neurosurgical clipping and endovascular coiling, which should be considered in dialogue between neurosurgery and neurointervention.
- Coiling has been associated with better outcomes in lower-grade SAH and is usually the preferred option when feasible.
- Whichever intervention is used, it should be performed as soon as possible, ideally within 72 hours.

- Hydrocephalus: in patients with radiological evidence of hydrocephalus and blood in the third or fourth ventricles, an external ventricular drain (EVD) is inserted, which can be used to reduce and drain pressure, and remove blood.

INTRACEREBRAL HAEMORRHAGE

In contrast to subarachnoid haemorrhage, an intracerebral haemorrhage is caused by bleeding into the brain tissue itself. Non-traumatic cases may be caused by systemic hypertension, damaged blood vessels or congenital abnormalities, such as an arteriovenous malformation (AVM).

Previous fit and well patients with a primary intracerebral haemorrhage accompanied by hydrocephalus should be considered for neurosurgical intervention. Patients with any of the following should be managed medically, although neurosurgical discussion is mandatory:

- Small, deep haemorrhages
- Lobar haemorrhages without hydrocephalus or rapid neurological deterioration
- A large haemorrhage with significant pre-existing co-morbidities
- A GCS of 8 or below unless caused by hydrocephalus
- Posterior fossa haemorrhage

Patients who are anticoagulated should have this reversed rapidly by administration of clotting factors and vitamin K.

ISCHAEMIC STROKE IN NEUROCRITICAL CARE

Traditionally associated with poor outcomes and a pessimistic view amongst clinicians regarding the prospects of neurological recovery, the management of acute ischaemic stroke has generally been delivered outside of the critical care unit. However, currently evolving interventional strategies have been shown to significantly improve outcome, and therefore such patients will be encountered increasingly more frequently on the neurocritical care unit in the future.

Acute ischaemic stroke is caused by occlusion of one or more of the cerebral arteries by a thrombus or embolism. Thrombolysis, the administration of systemic drugs in order to degrade clot, is commonplace within emergency departments in the United Kingdom, but does carry a significant risk of harm and the benefits are unclear.

Mechanical clot retrieval, also known as thrombectomy, is a relatively new technique employed by interventional neuroradiologists, which aims to remove the offending thrombus and restore blood flow and oxygen delivery to the affected brain tissue, thereby minimising brain damage. Eligible patients with a strong clinical suspicion of acute ischaemic stroke should have a plain CT and a CT/MR angiogram to confirm the presence of a thrombus immediately on admission to the hospital. The procedure involves insertion of a clot-retrieval device via the femoral artery to the occlusion site using X-ray guidance. The clot-retrieval device usually consists of a self-expanding metal mesh, which is partially deployed within the clot, traps it and is then withdrawn through the insertion catheter. Clot retrieval is sometimes accompanied by targeted arterial thrombolysis.

Although the optimum time interval between onset of symptoms and clot retrieval is unclear, outcomes seem to be better the sooner the procedure is performed, and an arbitrary eight-hour window has been advised at the time of writing this book.

Benefits shown in mechanical clot retrieval, compared to medical therapy alone include

- Reduction in mortality
- Improved revascularisation
- Improved 90-day functional independence
- Improved quality of life

Risks associated with the procedure include

- Embolisation of clot into distant vascular territories
- New ischaemic stroke in different vascular territories
- Cerebral vasospasm
- Cerebral vessel dissection and perforation
- Damage to access vessels, which may present as visible groin haemorrhage or occult retroperitoneal haemorrhage
- Contrast allergy

As with any primary brain injury, the general principle of neurocritical care is to minimise secondary brain injury by optimising blood flow to a swollen brain within the non-expansile skull. This is achieved by

- Mechanical factors: avoiding hard neck collars and ties on the ET tube, maintaining neutral head position and 30 degree head-up position. These improve venous drainage from the brain and reduce the intracranial pressure.
- Maintain a pO_2 of around 13 kPa and $PaCO_2$ of 4.5–5 kPa: hypoxia and hypercapnia will cause cerebral vasodilation, increasing the volume of intracranial blood and therefore intracranial pressure. Conversely, hypocapnia will cause vasoconstriction and reduced blood flow to already damaged brain tissue.
- Normoglycaemia.
- Normothermia: pyrexia, common in brain injuries, leads to an increased cerebral metabolic rate of oxygen demand, and will exacerbate any problem with oxygen delivery.
- Blood pressure: generally a mean arterial pressure of 90 mmHg is advised to maintain cerebral perfusion in brain injuries.
- Normovolaemia: whilst hypovolaemia will lead to problems with hypotension, hypervolaemia may conversely contribute to cerebral oedema and increased intracranial pressure.

DECOMPRESSIVE HEMICRANIECTOMY

A *malignant MCA infarct* is a term used to describe a middle cerebral artery (MCA) infarct, which leads to cerebral oedema and subsequent raised ICP, which compromises the blood supply to viable brain tissue and causes rapid neurological deterioration. Because some of the neurological deficit may be reversible, a subset of patients should be considered for a decompressive hemicraniectomy. By removing part of the fixed cranium and allowing the swollen brain to herniate through the defect, the aim is to reduce the pressure on blood vessels and restore flow to non-infarcted tissue. The following patients should be considered for this intervention:

- Aged up to 60
- Have clinical signs of an MCA territory infarct, with a National Institutes of Health Stroke Score (NIHSS) of more than 15
- Reduced level of consciousness
- CT evidence of infarct of more than 50% of the MCA territory, with or without infarct in the anterior or posterior cerebral artery territories, or infarct volume of more than 145 cm^3 on MR scan

Patients should be referred to the neurosurgical specialty within 24 hours of symptom onset, and the intervention performed within 48 hours.

WHAT DO YOU DO IN RESPONSE TO THE NURSE'S QUESTION? (ASSESSMENT OF PATIENT WITH DETERIORATING CONSCIOUS LEVEL AFTER DIAGNOSIS OF GRADE I SAH)

IMMEDIATE MANAGEMENT

As in all acute situations: an ABCDE approach ensures a structured approach.

1. Protect the airway if clinically indicated, with a cuffed endotracheal tube below the level of the vocal cords. Loss of airway-protective reflexes and vomiting associated with SAH are a recipe for aspiration pneumonia, which is a predictor of worse outcomes. The patient will likely require intra- or inter-hospital transfer and airway control is the first step in preparing for this.

2. If the patient requires mechanical ventilation, aim for a pO_2 of 13 kPa and $PaCO_2$ of 4.5–5 kPa to optimise their cerebral blood flow and ICP. Arterial cannulation for serial blood gas analysis and haemodynamic monitoring is essential.

3. Make sure there is adequate venous access. Discontinue antihypertensives. Aim to maintain systolic BP below 180 mmHg, with good analgesia, sedation and labetalol if needed. The mean arterial pressure (MAP) should be above 90 mmHg and use of vasopressors may be required.

4. Formally assess the GCS, pupil size and reactivity, and focal neurological deficit, and compare these to previously documented scores.

   Discuss at the earliest with the neurosurgical team about the deterioration once the patient is stabilised, seeking advice regarding urgent investigations, treatment and need for transfer to a tertiary neurosurgical centre.

   An urgent repeat CT brain scan if advised by the neurosurgical team should be performed without delay looking for possible early rebleed or hydrocephalus. Continue your dialogue with the neurosurgical team once the CT scan has been performed.

   Use an insulin infusion in the case of hyperglycaemia. Manage pyrexia with paracetamol +/– a cooling blanket. Treat clinically apparent seizures with anticonvulsant therapy according to local protocol.

Once stable, commence nimodipine 60 mg four-hourly orally. This will necessitate a nasogastric tube in the intubated patient. Nimodipine may cause transient hypotension, which should respond to fluids +/– vasopressors. It may be administered 30 mg two-hourly if hypotension is a problem.

5. Insert a urinary catheter if not already in situ, with hourly outputs measured. Prescribe graduated compression stockings and pneumatic devices unless contraindicated.

KEY LEARNING POINTS

- SAH is a potentially devastating neurological event with a 50%–60% mortality rate and carries a high risk of severe disability.
- Good basic critical care and timely, appropriate neurosurgical/neuroradiological intervention have a positive impact on patients' future lives.
- The most reliable predictor of outcome is neurological status on admission to hospital, which therefore forms the basis of the WFNS classification system.
- Eighty-five per cent of non-traumatic cases of SAH are caused by rupture of a cerebral aneurysm, which should be secured as soon as it is feasibly possible by clipping or coiling in order to prevent rebleeding.
- In addition to neurointervention, astute critical care, such as airway protection, neuroprotective ventilation, blood pressure control and prophylactic nimodipine amongst others, can optimise future neurological recovery in cases of SAH.
- Patients with ischaemic infarcts may undergo neurosurgical or neuroradiology intervention and subsequently are cared for on neurocritical care.

FURTHER READING

National Confidential Enquiry into Patient Outcome and Death (NCEPOD). "Subarachnoid Haemorrhage: Managing the Flow." 2013. www.ncepod.org.uk/2013sah.html (accessed 10 May 2017).

National Institute for Health and Care Excellence (NICE). *Mechanical Clot Retrieval for Treating Acute Ischaemic Stroke*. Interventional Procedures Guidance IPG548, National Institute for Health and Care Excellence, Manchester, UK, February 2016. www.nice.org.uk/guidance/ipg548 (accessed 12 May 2017).

National Institute for Health and Care Excellence (NICE). *Stroke and Transient Ischaemic Attack in over 16s: Diagnosis and Initial Management*. Clinical Guideline 68, National Institute for Health and Care Excellence, Manchester, UK, July 2008 (updated March 2017). www.nice.org.uk/guidance/cg68 (accessed 14 May 2017).

Steiner, Thorsten, Seppo Juvela, Andreas Unterberg, Carla Jung, Michael Forsting, and Gabriel Rinkel. "European Stroke Organization Guidelines for the Management of Intracranial Aneurysms and Subarachnoid Haemorrhage." *Cerebrovascular Diseases* 35 (February 2013): 93–112.

46

Ongoing management of the patient with burns

KAREN MEACHER AND THOMAS OWEN

'Could you assess Bed 3? I think he's developing an infection.'

Patients with significant or complicated burn injuries are cared for in specialist burn centres where an experienced multidisciplinary team ensures that all aspects of care address the specific needs of this challenging group of patients.

This chapter is intended as a brief overview of the ways in which patients with burn injuries differ from other patient populations. The days following resuscitation of a patient with a burn injury are marked by the significant systemic response to the release of inflammatory mediators, resulting in hypermetabolism and immunosuppression, as well as complications specific to the burn injury itself.

SYSTEMIC CONSIDERATIONS

CARDIOVASCULAR

- Increased capillary permeability resulting in tissue oedema
- Myocardial depression
- Peripheral and splanchnic vasoconstriction

RESPIRATORY

- Bronchoconstriction due to inflammatory mediators
- ARDS in presence of smoke inhalation injury

GENITOURINARY TRACT

- High calorific requirements (up to double normal) necessitate supplementary enteral nutrition.
- Increased risk of GI stress ulcers, need ulcer prophylaxis.
- Risk of abdominal compartment syndrome.
- Risk of faecal contamination of lower limb and perineal wounds.

RENAL

- At risk of injury due to multiple causes, e.g. sepsis, rhabdomyolysis, abdominal compartment syndrome

NEUROLOGICAL

- Procedural pain (dressing changes) and background pain
- Development of neuropathic pain (hyperalgesia)
- Hypoxic brain injury sustained due to confinement at scene (hypoxic environment) or carbon monoxide toxicity

MUSCULOSKELETAL

- Loss of function in limbs affected by burns
- Risk of compartment syndrome

ELECTROLYTE

- Increased loss of Na^+ and Cl^- in exudate fluid
- Hypophosphataemia common in first few days
- Suxamethonium contraindicated from 48 hours to 1 year post injury due to risk of hyperkalaemia

METABOLISM

- Increase in basal metabolic rate proportional to size of burn, resulting in catabolism
- Hypercatabolic/hypermetabolic state driven by catecholamine and cortisol release
- Can persist for up to 2 years post injury
- Patient's baseline core temperature reset to 38.5°C

HAEMATOLOGICAL

- Severe burns associated with haemolysis and disseminated intravascular coagulation (DIC)

IMMUNE

- Suppressed immune response
- Disruption of barrier function of skin

PSYCHOLOGICAL

- Depression and anxiety (multifactorial)
- Post-traumatic stress disorder
- Increased ICU (intensive care unit) delirium risk due to high sedative and analgesia requirements
- Sleep disturbance

SPECIFIC CONSIDERATIONS

SMOKE INHALATION INJURY

Patients who have been intubated because of smoke inhalation require specific care and management considerations:

- Uncut ETT needs to be marked at the teeth, and correct position should be confirmed daily due to risk of facial and airway swelling causing dislodgment of tube.
- Lung protective ventilation strategies (V_T 6–7 mL/kg, P_{INSP} < 30 cmH$_2$O, PEEP as required).
- Patients with carbon monoxide poisoning should be ventilated with FiO$_2$ 1.0 until carboxyhaemoglobin levels (COHb) have normalised.
- Regular therapeutic bronchoscopy with lavage may be indicated if soot deposits are found on following initial diagnostic bronchoscopy.
- Regular chest physiotherapy to encourage mobilisation of secretions.
- Patients will require saline and salbutamol nebulisers.
- Nebulised mucolytics may be considered (N-acetylcysteine and heparin).
- Oral mucolytic (carbocysteine) may also be given.
- Patients are vulnerable to ventilator associated pneumonia (VAP); high index of suspicion needed.

BURN SHOCK, FLUID RESUSCITATION AND MANAGEMENT

As mentioned in Chapter 16 on acute management of burns, during the first 24–48 hours, there is massive fluid shift and fluid loss resulting in hypovolaemic shock. Various fluid regimens have been devised to estimate the volume of fluid that these patients need, of which the Parkland formula is a well-known example.

Patients may not have received their calculated fluid amounts prior to transfer, or the extent of their burn injury may have been underestimated and so they have been undertreated. Alternatively, 'fluid creep' may have occurred, and the patient may have given too much fluid or too quickly, leading to increased oedema formation and increased risk of abdominal compartment syndrome.

Specialist burn centres will have their own local guidelines for fluid resuscitation and management, using a mix of crystalloid and colloid fluids. The general aim is for a urine output of 0.5–1.0 mL/kg/hr as an indication of adequate volume resuscitation. However, particularly unstable patients may require cardiac output monitoring and inotropic support. Seek senior assistance if you feel this is indicated.

TEMPERATURE REGULATION

Patients are at risk of hypothermia due to a combination of the failure of the thermoregulating properties of skin, and heat loss via evaporation from wounds. In addition, they enter into a hypermetabolic state and their base line core temperature increases. Our usual definition of normothermia (36°C–37.5°C) is considered hypothermia in a burn patient. They should be nursed in an elevated temperature environment with active warming as required, and core temperature should be closely monitored and maintained at around 37.5°C–38.5°C. They may require active cooling if their core temperature exceeds 40°C despite antipyretics and simple cooling measures (e.g. cold IV fluid, fan).

WOUND INFECTION/SEPSIS

Patients become immunocompromised following significant burn injuries:

- Loss of skin (a significant part of the host defence)
- Raised cortisol levels from stress response, causing immunosuppression
- Reduced lymphocyte activity (multifactorial)

The majority of normal skin flora is destroyed (obviously!) in the area of skin that is burned, but reservoirs in sweat glands and hair follicles mean that *Staphylococcus* and other Gram-positive organisms recolonise the burn wound surface in the 48 hours following injury. These wounds are protein-rich environments filled with necrotic tissue, and over the next week they are joined by a mix of Gram-positive and Gram-negative microbes. Over time, especially with exposure to broad-spectrum antibiotics, fungal species may start to predominate.

However, this is wound *colonisation*, not wound *infection*. Antibiotics should never be started because of a positive swab culture; instead, look for evidence of localised or systemic infection:

- Offensive odour from wound
- Increasing oedema or cellulitis, or advancement of necrotic tissue
- Fever > 39°C or hypothermia < 36.5°C
- Rising white cell count (WCC)
- Tachycardia > 110 bpm or increasing inotrope/vasopressor requirements
- Worsening tachypnoea > 25/min or increasing FiO_2 requirements
- Thrombocytopaenia
- New hyperglycaemia
- New diarrhoea or failure to absorb enteral feed (gut failure)

Full cultures should be performed (peripheral, line, wound swabs, sputum, urine, etc.) and microbiology advice sought as to appropriate antibiotic therapy.

47

Ageing and frailty

VANISHA PATEL AND JOYCE YEUNG

Mrs Smith is an 83-year-old lady admitted with severe community-acquired pneumonia. She has a background history of angina, hypertension and chronic obstructive pulmonary disease (COPD). She lives alone but her daughter has mentioned a decline in her health and she has been struggling to cope at home over the last few months.

What are the important issues to assess and discuss for this elderly patient in relation to critical care admission?

THE AGEING POPULATION

Globally the population is ageing and currently in the United Kingdom there are 11.6 million people over 65 years of age and 1.5 million aged over 80. The Office of National Statistics predicts that by 2040 nearly one in four (24.2%) people in the United Kingdom will be aged over 65 years. Emergency cases account for 14,000 admissions per year to intensive care in England and Wales. The mortality of these cases is over 25% and the intensive care unit (ICU) cost alone is at least £88 million. Our ageing population will have a significant impact on public-health service resources.

THE ELDERLY – THE CHALLENGES

As patients age, there is an accompanying physiological decline, the presence of multiple comorbidities, polypharmacy and frailty. This coupled with an acute illness and admission to critical care can lead to both short- and long-term adverse outcomes. Identifying which of these patients will benefit most from critical care is therefore a challenge facing critical care physicians. Of note, it is well recognised that age alone is a poor predictor of outcome.

PHYSIOLOGICAL AND PATHOLOGICAL CHANGES ASSOCIATED WITH THE ELDERLY

- After the age of 40, there is approximately a 1% reduction in organ reserve per year. Loss of physiological reserve leads to the reduced capacity for organs to cope with superimposed stressors of an acute illness or surgery.

CARDIOVASCULAR

- Myocardial fibrosis and ventricular wall stiffening (diastolic dysfunction) leads to a reduction in cardiac compliance and cardiac output. As a result, the cardiovascular system has a reduced capacity to cope with stress due to a reduction in baroreceptor sensitivity and an increased risk of hypotension and a requirement for higher doses of inotropes.
- Cardiac atherosclerosis can lead to myocardial ischaemia.
- Dysrhythmias are common including atrial fibrillation.

RESPIRATORY

- Lung function declines due to reduced lung and chest wall compliance.
- There is a decreased sensitivity of the respiratory centre to hypoxia and hypercapnia leading to an increased risk of respiratory failure.
- There is loss of alveolar gas exchange surface.
- Age-related decline in oxidative capacity can lead to an increased risk of myocardial and cerebral ischaemia.

RENAL

- Reduction in renal tissue mass and glomeruli leads to a decline in renal function.
- There is deterioration in renal tubular function and a decreased ability to clear renally excreted drugs.
- The nephrotoxic effects of diseases (hypertension, diabetes) and drugs (NSAIDS, ACE inhibitors) can lead to renal failure.

NEUROLOGICAL

- There is a reduction in neuronal mass and density leading to decreased sympathetic and parasympathetic responsiveness.
- There is an increased risk of syncope, strokes, gait and visual disturbances.
- Age-related decline in cerebral and cardiovascular function can lead to delirium or cognitive dysfunction, which delays recovery.

HAEMATOLOGICAL

- Anaemia is common and is thought to be due to erythropoietin resistance or 'stem cell ageing'.
- Increased risk of hypercoagulability increases the risk of developing deep vein thrombosis.

MUSCULOSKELETAL

- Sarcopaenia – The reduction in muscle volume and function, thinning skin and immobility accelerates the development of pressure sores.

NUTRITION

- Malnutrition is common amongst hospitalised elderly patients and it is associated with adverse outcomes.
- Enteral nutrition over parenteral nutrition improves outcome.
- Protein supplementation may ameliorate the effects of sarcopaenia.

PHARMACOLOGICAL

- There is variation in pharmacokinetics and pharmacodynamics.
- The elimination half-life of drugs such as opioids and benzodiazepines is increased due to reduced renal and hepatic blood flow.
- Due to a smaller blood volume and reduced protein binding, there is a higher free-drug concentration.
- Due to polypharmacy, there is an increased risk of drug interactions.

FUNCTIONAL DECLINE

- Following a period of bed-rest or immobility, elderly patients can experience deconditioning. This is a multi-factorial, physiological process leading to a decline in mental ability, continence and functional ability in activities of daily living; it is common amongst patients admitted with an acute illness. A reduction in functional ability can lead to long-term disability particularly in the frail elderly patient.

FRAILTY AND FRAILTY ASSESSMENT

Frailty is a widely used term describing the state of vulnerability that puts a patient at increased risk of morbidity and mortality. It is thought to affect approximately 25% of patients aged over 85 years and can be defined as 'a medical syndrome with multiple causes and contributors that is characterized by diminished strength, endurance, and reduced physiologic function that increases an individual's vulnerability for developing increased dependency and/or death' (Morley, 2013).

Frailty can be associated with disease, lack of activity and mobility, poor nutrition, stress and the physiological changes associated with ageing. It is a recognised determinant of morbidity, mortality and long-term outcomes such as increasing disability and institutionalisation.

Two main theoretical constructs exist in frailty assessment, the phenotypic model or the deficit model (Fried et al., 2001; Mitnitski et al., 2001).

- Fried et al.'s phenotypic model defines five components: exhaustion, weight loss, weak grip strength, slow walking speed and low physical activity. The presence of three suggests multi-system dysregulation and frailty.
- The deficit model calculates accumulated deficits over a lifetime; it recognises frailty as a multidimensional index not based purely on physical status. It is a multi-domain phenotype that determines deficits in physical, cognitive, functional and social aspects of a patient's life. The Canadian Study of Health and Aging (CSHA) developed a 70-item frailty index (FI). The index was calculated by dividing the number of items present in a patient divided by 70 (the total number of variables being measured). The FI calculated was found to be able to predict survival.

A modified nine-point clinical frailty scale (CFS) based on judgement has been subsequently developed and validated. It comprises nine discrete categories ranging from vey fit to terminally ill. The CFS has been recognised to predict mortality and institutionalisation in critical care. Although other models exist, the CFS is simple and easy to use on patients that are acutely unwell to determine their prehospital frailty status.

PROGNOSTIC IMPLICATIONS

Frailty assessment provides additional prognostic value to clinicians in decisions surrounding appropriateness of an intensive care admission, withholding of life-sustaining treatment and end-of-life care decision-making. It can facilitate discussions with patients/relatives around appropriate treatment options, prognosis and decisions regarding escalation of treatment and resuscitation.

The use of a frailty index as an assessment tool in critical care is an evolving concept. Frailty is a common pre-existing state for patients in critical care. The use of frailty scoring in predicting short- and long-term outcomes has been found to be superior to using chronological age alone.

Studies have shown a frailty to be a cause of longer length of stay in intensive care and total hospitalisation (Bagshaw, 2014). However, longer-term outcomes, such as disability, quality of life and function, have not been investigated.

The advantage of using an FI as a prognostic tool is that it takes into account the burden of co-morbid diseases, pre-hospital functional status and disability that other risk adjustment tools, such as the Acute Physiology and Chronic Health Evaluation (APACHE II), Sequential Organ Failure Assessment (SOFA) and Simplified Acute Physiology Score (SAPS) systems, do not necessarily do.

When an elderly patient leaves critical care, the rehabilitation issues are more complex than that of a young patient. Ability to return home, adequate quality of life and independence are important prognostic features for the elderly.

THERAPEUTIC IMPLICATIONS

A multi-dimensional approach to reduce the progression of frailty has been sought. These include physical, nutritional and psychological therapies to reduce adverse outcomes for frail patients. Currently, nutritional support, early physiotherapy and sedation holds are part of the daily assessment of patients on critical care.

In the critical care environment, following identification and stratification of this population, the development of a multi-faceted intervention to target the frailty cycle represents an area for future research.

BACK TO THE CASE

What are the important issues to assess and discuss for this patient in relation to admission to critical care? Admission to critical care for the elderly should not be based on chronological age alone but following review and discussion surrounding the following criteria:

1. Initial assessment and timely resuscitation
   a. An initial ABCDE assessment
   b. Supportive treatment including oxygen therapy, intravenous fluids, antibiotics and sepsis management
2. Severity of acute illness
   a. Review of the clinical history including the course of the acute illness as well as any deterioration in general health in the lead-up to this hospital admission
3. ICU admission criteria
   a. Assessment of co-morbidities and chronic illness and the impact of these on organ function. For example, if a patient is known to have diabetes, are there any macro- or micro-vascular complications reducing physiological reserve of an organ system?
   b. Functional status including mobility, exercise tolerance; are they independent of activities of daily living or are they housebound and rely on family/carers to help wash/dress/do their shopping?
4. Frailty and disability assessment and risk prediction
   a. Review of pre-hospital frailty and disability status to guide prognosis of outcomes
5. Impact of treatment on outcome
   a. Treatments and procedures are commenced with the intention of achieving beneficial outcomes that are perceived to be important by patients. However, these can be invasive and harmful; therefore, review of appropriate procedures, therapies and interventions should occur.
6. Discussion with patients +/- their carers/relatives, including expression of wishes regarding escalating treatment and resuscitation
   a. Patient's wishes together with those of their relatives/carers should be taken into account when considering critical care admission.
   b. Limitations or withdrawal of treatment and end of life care should be discussed early when appropriate.
   c. An advanced directive or power of attorney should be identified if relevant.

7. Early involvement of the multi-disciplinary team
   a. Early involvement of dietician support, physiotherapy to aid early mobilisation
   b. Care of the Elderly Consultant input to facilitate early rehabilitation

---

KEY LEARNING POINTS

- The elderly are a challenging cohort of patients presenting with multiple co-morbidities, poly-pharmacy, frailty and disability.
- Physiological and pathological organ decline is common.
- Frailty assessment can provide an additional risk prediction tool to inform patients, their carers/relatives and physicians to guide management.
- Early shared decision making between patients and their carers/relatives and clinicians is advocated.

FURTHER READING

Bagshaw, Sean M., H. Thomas Stelfox, Robert C. McDermid, Darryl B. Rolfson, Ross T. Tsuyuki, Nadia Baig, Barbara Artiuch, Quazi Ibrahim, Daniel E. Stollery, Ella Rokosh, and Sumit R. Majumdar. "Association Between Frailty and Short- and Long-Term Outcomes Among Critically Ill Patients: A Multicentre Prospective Cohort Study." *Canadian Medical Association Journal* 186, no. 2 (February 2014): E95–E102.

Fried, Linda P., Catherine M. Tangen, Jeremy Walston, Anne B. Newman, Calvin Hirsch, John Gottdiener, Teresa Seeman, Russell Tracy, Willem J. Kop, Gregory Burke, and Mary Ann McBurnie for the Cardiovascular Health Study Collaborative Research Group. "Frailty in Older Adults: Evidence for a Phenotype." *The Journals of Gerontology, Series A, Biological Sciences and Medical Sciences* 56A, no. 3 (2001): M146–M156.

Griffiths, Richard, Fiona Beech, Alan Brown, Jugdeep Dhesi, Irwin Foo, Jonathan Goodall, William Harrop-Griffiths, John Jameson, Nick Love, Karin Pappenheim, and Stuart White. "Peri-Operative Care of the Elderly 2014: Association of Anaesthetists of Great Britain and Ireland." *Anaesthesia.* 69, suppl. 1 (January 2014): 81–98.

Heyland, Daren K., Allan Garland, Sean M. Bagshaw, Deborah Cook, Kenneth Rockwood, Henry T. Stelfox, Peter Dodek, Robert A. Fowler, Alexis F. Turgeon, Karen Burns, John Muscedere, Jim Kutsogiannis, Martin Albert, Sangeeta Mehta, Xuran Jiang, and Andrew G. Day. "Recovery After Critical Illness in Patients Aged 80 Years or Older: A Multi-Center Prospective Observational Cohort Study." *Intensive Care Medicine* 41, no. 11 (November 2015): 1911–1920.

Mitnitski, Arnold B., Alexander J. Mogilner, and Kenneth Rockwood. "Accumulation of Deficits As a Proxy Measure of Aging." *The Scientific World Journal* 1 (August 2001): 323–336.

Morley, John E., Bruno Vellas, G. Abellan van Kan, Stefan D. Anker, Juergen M. Bauer, Roberto Bernabei, Matteo Cesari, W.C. Chumlea, Wolfram Doehner, Jonathan Evans, Linda P. Fried, Jack M. Guralnik, Paul R. Katz, Theodore K. Malmstrom, Roger J. McCarter, Luis M. Gutierrez Robledo, Ken Rockwood, Stephan von Haehling, Maurits F. Vandewoude, and Jeremy Walston. "Frailty Consensus: A Call to Action." *Journal of the American Medical Directors Association* 14, no. 6 (June 2013): 392–397.

48

Transfer of the critically ill patient

EMMA FOSTER AND NEIL CROOKS

Mr Smith is a 25-year-old man who has been admitted to the ICU following a head injury that resulted in an acute subdural haematoma. He was intubated on arrival in the Emergency Department (ED) for a low Glasgow Coma Scale (GCS) and had an intracranial pressure (ICP) monitor inserted prior to arrival in the ICU. His ICP has now increased and his pupils have become unequal. You discuss the case with the neurosurgical team who ask for a repeat CT scan of the head. You are asked to transfer him safely for this scan. How do you do this?

INTRODUCTION

A critical care transfer is the movement of any critically ill patient either within a hospital *(intra-hospital transfer)* or to another hospital *(inter-hospital transfer)* so the patient can receive definitive care from a specialist team. Non-clinical or capacity transfers may take place when the only critical care resource is available at another location. The aim of an effective transfer is to provide on-going critical care support in a safe manner, despite the environmental change.

All critical care transfers are associated with a degree of risk due to complications arising from the transfer. This includes deterioration in the patient's clinical condition, as critically ill patients tend to tolerate movement and environmental change poorly. These transfers should be undertaken by staff with appropriate competencies, qualifications and experience with senior clinicians involved in the decision-making process. However, many ICUs in the United Kingdom will only be involved in a small number of transfers each year, and individual staff will lack transfer experience. This has led the Intensive Care Society to recommend the introduction of specialist retrieval teams who can be mobilised from the receiving hospital to transfer the patient. However, these are yet to fully evolve in the UK adult ICU setting (Table 48.1).

Table 48.1 Categories of critical care transfers in the United Kingdom

Categories of transfers	
Primary	Movement of a patient from a pre-hospital site to the immediate receiving hospital
Secondary	Movement of a patient between any two hospitals
Tertiary	Transfer of a patient from a secondary or tertiary hospital to a national centre of expertise
Quaternary	International transfers

PREPARATION FOR TRANSFER

The decision to transfer a patient must be carefully weighed against the risks and benefits. Each case should be assessed individually with regards to stability, need for and timing of transfer along with the skill mix required to carry out the transfer safely and manage any complications *en route*. Intensivists in the referring and receiving hospitals would normally take this decision in conjunction with colleagues from the relevant specialities involved in the patient's care. Complications arising during a transfer can be particularly difficult to manage due to the limited access to the patient and constraints of the transport environment. Therefore, thorough preparation is essential and the use of checklists is mandatory.

The ABCDE approach is one method that can be used for the assessment, planning and preparation of the patient for transfer. This should be used in conjunction with a checklist to ensure that all aspects of the patient's care are considered.

AIRWAY (WITH CERVICAL SPINE IMMOBILISATION IF INDICATED)

- Patients at risk of airway compromise should be intubated prior to transfer
- The endotracheal (ET) tube should be well secured. Size, length, grade of laryngoscopy at intubation recorded
- Chest radiograph confirming ET tube position
- Tracheostomy tube – size, cuff, fenestration, date of insertion, inner tube present
- Capnography
- Face mask and airway adjuncts
- Self-inflating (Ambu®) bag
- Water's circuit (Remember this requires an oxygen supply!)
- Appropriate range of airway equipment (e.g. laryngoscopes)

A plan should be in place for any airway complications, e.g. displaced ET or tracheostomy tube. You must consider how you would maintain the airway and what equipment you would need if such a situation were to arise, e.g. bag mask ventilation, airway adjuncts and face mask, possibility of re-intubation or reinsertion of tracheostomy tube.

BREATHING

- Record baseline oxygen requirement, minute ventilation and oxygen saturations.
- Portable ventilator
  - Ensure that the team is familiar with the ventilator and that safety checks are completed.
  - Set the portable ventilator based on current parameters.
  - Ensure ventilation is adequate and patient stable on the portable ventilator for approximately ten minutes prior to departure.
- Arterial blood gas (ABG) – Prior to transfer, this will give an indication of stability of the patient and adequacy of ventilation.
- Ability to continue ventilation in event of ventilator failure.
  - Ambu® bag
  - Waters circuit
- Stethoscope.
- Intercostal drain (if present) attached to Heimlich valve.
- Oxygen.
  - Adequate supplies (oxygen calculation) in vehicle and portable cylinders
- Oxygen Consumption
  - Total volume of oxygen required (L) = 2 × (minute volume (L) × bias flow (L)) × duration of transfer in minutes
  - This is multiplied by 2 to allow for delays *en route*.
  - Assumes FiO_2 of 1.0 in case patient deteriorates.
  - The bias flow is any additional oxygen flow required to drive the ventilator. This will normally be displayed on the ventilator.

CIRCULATION

- Examine cardiovascular system and record baseline observations.
- Adequate intravenous (IV) access? Minimum access is two peripheral cannulae. Determine which is your closest access for drug administration. Are they secured?
- Is the patient haemodynamically stable?
- Adequate haemoglobin concentration?

- ECG and invasive blood pressure (IBP) monitoring, with non-invasive blood pressure (NIBP) monitoring as backup. Invasive BP monitoring is less sensitive to movement artefact.
- Drugs
  - Any vasopressor or inotropic support required?
  - Sufficient quantities available for transfer plus delays.
  - Additional emergency drugs, e.g. metaraminol, adrenaline, vagolytics.
  - Fluids – 1 L crystalloid run through a giving set and attached to the patient.

DISABILITY

- Baseline GCS (if not sedated) and pupil size and reaction.
- If a transferring a spinal injury patient, ensure there is documentation of current neurology to allow for monitoring of changes *en route*.
- Adequate sedation for the transfer allowing for delays?
- It usually appropriate to fully sedate and paralyse the patient for the transfer.
- Blood glucose (> 4.0 mmol/L).
- If insulin infusion is running, may be pragmatic to temporarily discontinue for a short transfer (and any other non-essential infusions, e.g. parenteral nutrition).
- Head injury patients – Osmotic diuretic (e.g. mannitol).

EVERYTHING ELSE

- Nasogastric tube – reduces risk of regurgitation, decompresses stomach (important on aeromedical transfers)
- Urinary catheter in situ – bag emptied prior to departure
- Investigations
  - Imaging – hard copies of relevant reports and transfer of scans to receiving hospital
  - Pathology/microbiology/drug charts
- Equipment and monitoring
  - Equipment should be portable and certified for transport use.
  - Batteries should be charged with sufficient life for the duration of the transfer.

- Appropriate alarm limits should be set prior to transfer.
- The minimum monitoring set of ECG, BP, SPO_2 and $EtCO_2$ should be maintained throughout the transfer.
- Ideally, a bespoke transfer trolley will be used for the movement of critically ill patients. These trolleys are specially designed to securely store all the necessary equipment and will be British Standard 1789/2000 compliant.

- Environmental
  - Patient warming and temperature monitoring
  - Pressure area care (position changes may be required on longer transfers)
  - Patient and equipment secured
- Inter-hospital
  - Telephone number for receiving unit and pre-departure call
  - Communication of any complications or delays *en route*
  - Destination and access to receiving unit confirmed with driver
  - Appropriate clothing and footwear
  - Mobile phone and money
  - Plan for returning team to base

The Intensive Care Society has published detailed lists specifying the minimum drug and equipment requirements for transfers (*Guidelines for the Transport of the Critically Ill Adult*, 3rd edition, 2011).

SPECIAL CIRCUMSTANCES

Transfer medicine is a broad area of critical care medicine encompassing evacuation, repatriation and aeromedical work. Evacuation involves instituting critical care treatment before and during transfer of a patient to an appropriate hospital for ongoing critical care management. This may take place on the battlefield, following a trauma (e.g. road traffic accident) or from another country where the local medical facilities may be inadequate. Examples of this are Medical Emergency Response Teams (MERT), the regional HEMS (Helicopter Emergency Medical Service) organisations, and fixed wing air ambulance providers, e.g. Air Alliance Medflight UK. Repatriation is a non-emergent process, which usually takes place when the patient is in the recovery phase of their illness and is deemed safe to travel back to their country of origin. It is usually funded by insurance companies and involves flying a team to a foreign country to assesses and transfer the patient.

Retrievals usually involve a specialist team travelling to a hospital in order to assess, stabilise and subsequently transfer a patient to a specialist centre. This is used in the United Kingdom for most paediatric critical care transfers. This is also the model used for many adult critical care transfers in Australia and New Zealand. These countries both have a low population density and the specialist medical care is centred in large hospitals; therefore, patients may have to travel long distances for medical care. This arrangement has led to the development of organisations such as the Royal Flying Doctor Service.

Aeromedical work involves the use of either fixed-wing or rotary-wing aircraft. The choice of which will depend on the weather conditions, time of day, distance, urgency of transfer and underlying clinical problem.

AEROMEDICAL TRANSFERS

Aeromedical transfers impose the physiological changes that occur with acceleration, deceleration, change in ambient pressure, noise and vibration on the critically ill patient. Boyle's law states that there is volume expansion with decreasing pressure. Therefore, gas in body cavities will expand as cabin pressure decreases, e.g. bowel obstruction, pneumothorax and pneumocephalus. This may necessitate insertion of intercostal drains, nasogastric tube or pressurisation of the cabin to sea level. Pressure change at altitude will also affect equipment, e.g. pressure bags for invasive arterial blood pressure and endotracheal tube cuffs.

Dalton's law of partial pressures is another key principle in altitude physiology, as it describes how a reduction in pressure leads to a reduction in oxygen availability. In other words, if a patient is hypoxic at sea level, they will be even more hypoxic at altitude.

MRI

Transfer of ICU patients to MRI presents its own unique challenges. New MRI units should be equipped to accept ventilated patients, with a control room from where the patient can be monitored. Immediate access to the patient is essential to allow rapid extraction from the magnetic field in the event of sudden deterioration. All equipment in the scanning room must be MR safe or MR conditional, and guidelines on use should be adhered to and minimum monitoring standards should be followed.

CASE ANSWER

The key points with regard to transfer of the 25-year-old man in the clinical vignette are outlined below.

AIRWAY

- Intubated and ventilated, grade I intubation, size 8 ET tube tied at 22 cm.
- Spare ET tube sizes 8, 7.5 and 8.5.
- Laryngoscope, face mask, airway adjuncts, Ambu® bag and waters circuit.
- In event of accidental extubation, maintain airway and oxygenation with bag mask ventilation and an airway adjunct, with a view to re-intubation. Alternative strategy is insertion of a Laryngeal Mask Airway (LMA).

BREATHING

- SaO_2 98% on FiO_2 0.3, RR 14, SIMV on the portable ventilator with tidal volume set at 500 mL, PEEP 5, minute ventilation 7 L, and bias flow of 1 L, achieving satisfactory CO_2 clearance.
- Chest clear on auscultation with good air entry bilaterally.
- CXR confirms ET tube and central line in satisfactory positions.
- Oxygen required for a transfer time of one hour with a minute ventilation of 7 L and bias flow of 1 L = $2 \times 7.0 \times 1.0 \times 60 = 840$ L, therefore need a size F cylinder or $2 \times$ CD cylinders.

CIRCULATION

- BP 148/85, P 86, ECG = normal sinus rhythm, urinary catheter in situ with last three hours urine output of 60, 90, 160 mL/hr
- Haemodynamically stable
- Access – internal jugular central line, and a 16 g cannula in the right antecubital fossa
- Invasive monitoring in situ. Manual BP cuff attached
- Patient 0.2 mcg/kg/min noradrenaline to maintain a mean arterial BP with adequate amount for transfer

DISABILITY

- Left pupil size 6, right pupil size 3 – left non-reactive
- Sedated with propofol and alfentanil infusions with three hours remaining on infusions
- Spare syringe of infusions and emergency drugs to hand
- Paralysed with a non-depolarising muscle relaxant for transfer

EVERYTHING ELSE

- You have the notes and drugs chart with you.
- NG feeding and non-essential infusions discontinued.
- Appropriate team – experienced ICU nurse, porters.
- You have a mobile phone to contact consultant if there are any problems.

SUMMARY

Transfer of the critically ill patient presents logistical and clinical challenges, with the risk of deterioration away from immediate help. However, with experienced staff, appropriate equipment and meticulous preparation and planning, it is possible to minimise the risks and transfer these patients safely.

FURTHER READING

Ashton-Cleary, Dave, and Kelly Mackey. "Inter-Hospital Transfers." Anaesthesia Tutorial of the Week, Tutorial 319, World Federation of Societies of Anaesthesiologists, London, UK, August 2015.

Association of Anaesthetists of Great Britain and Ireland. "Provision of Anaesthetic Services in Magnetic Resonance Units." The Association of Anaesthetists of Great Britain and Ireland, London, May 2002.

Association of Anaesthetists of Great Britain and Ireland. "Interhospital Transfer." AAGBI Safety Guideline. The Association of Anaesthetists of Great Britain and Ireland, London, February 2009.

Droogh, Joep M., Marije Smit, Anthony R. Absalom, Jack J.M. Ligtenberg, and Jan G. Zijlstra. "Transferring the Critically Ill Patient: Are We There Yet?" *Critical Care* 19, no. 1 (February 2015): 62.

Intensive Care Society. *Guidelines for the Transport of the Critically Ill Adult.* 3rd ed. London: Intensive Care Society, 2011.

Low, Adam, and Jonathan Hulme, eds. *ABC of Transfer and Retrieval Medicine,* 1st ed. Chichester: Wiley-Blackwell, 2014.

49

The critically ill obstetric patient

JENNIFER HARES AND NARESH SANDUR

You are called to the Emergency Department resus citation room to review a 25-year-old lady. She is 23 weeks pregnant, gravida 2 para 1.

She gives a three-day history of worsening shortness of breath, abdominal pain and headache.

Since 2000, MBRRACE-UK (Mothers and Babies: Reducing Risk through Audits and Confidential Enquiries across the UK, formerly CMACH & CMACE) has investigated the causes of maternal death in the United Kingdom. They produce detailed reports, which include key points and lessons learned.

The information in this chapter focuses on the areas, which have been highlighted in the reports as important in improving the care of the sick obstetric patient.

DIFFERENTIAL DIAGNOSES

The diagnoses of particular importance are *highlighted in italics* and will be discussed in more detail later in this chapter.

SHORTNESS OF BREATH (SOB)

SOB is a common symptom, which can start in any trimester. It can be experienced by up to 75% of pregnant women (Centre for Maternal and Child Enquiries [CMACE], 2011).

ASTHMA

It is important never to assume that wheeze on auscultation represents asthma. Most women with asthma will have an established diagnosis before pregnancy. It is unusual for asthma to present for the first time in pregnancy.

A new wheeze could be pulmonary oedema (CMACE, 2011).

Red flags suggesting a more ominous underlying pathology include

- Sudden onset shortness of breath
- Associated with chest pain
- Orthopnoea or paroxysmal nocturnal dyspnoea (PND) (CMACE, 2011)

PULMONARY EMBOLUS

This classically presents with sudden onset breathlessness with associated pleuritic pain, haemoptysis and/or dizziness.

PNEUMONIA

The presentation of pneumonia in the obstetric patient is similar to the non-obstetric patient with cough, fever and raised inflammatory markers.

BACTERIAL PNEUMONIA

- Common pathogens include pneumococcal pneumonia and group A streptococcal pneumonia.

VIRAL PNEUMONIA

- Pregnant women are particularly susceptible to viral pneumonia such as H1N1, varicella zoster and influenza A & B.
- The recommendation is that early antiviral treatment should be instigated for pregnant women with a differential diagnosis of influenza (Knight et al., 2014).

Severe respiratory failure in pregnant women failing to respond to standard ventilatory support should be referred early to an ECMO centre (Knight et al., 2014).

PULMONARY OEDEMA

Pulmonary oedema usually presents with classical signs and symptoms such as orthopnoea, paroxysmal nocturnal dyspnoea (PND) and frothy/pink sputum. Fine inspiratory crackles and/or wheeze may be heard on auscultation. Pulmonary oedema may be due to:

- Fluid overload, especially in the context of *pre-eclampsia*
- Cardiac failure

PULMONARY ARTERIAL HYPERTENSION (PAH)

PAH is poorly tolerated in pregnancy and in particular during labour with a mortality rate of 30%–50% (Burt and Durbridge, 2009). Breathlessness may be the only symptom and often gets worse with exercise/labour.

It may be seen in conditions such as left heart disease, chronic lung disease and/or hypoxia and thromboembolism.

If PAH is suspected, a chest X-ray and echocardiography should be performed and oxygen saturations recorded.

These ladies need managing in an appropriate high-dependency unit (HDU) environment.

ABDOMINAL PAIN OR DIARRHOEA AND VOMITING

PRE-CONCEPTION

- Ovarian Hyperstimulation Syndrome (OHSS)
  OHSS is a complication of ovarian stimulation fertility treatment. Although rare, the incidence is increasing as the access to fertility treatment becomes more widespread.

Local and systemic pro-inflammatory mediators cause vascular permeability, which can result in ascites, pulmonary and/or pericardial effusions. Severe cases can present with hypovolaemia, thromboembolism and adult respiratory distress syndrome (Royal College of Obstetricians and Gynaecologists, 2016).

IN EARLY PREGNANCY

- Ectopic pregnancy can occur in the absence of vaginal bleeding. A diagnosis of ectopic pregnancy should be considered in all women of childbearing age presenting with hypotension sufficient to cause fainting and dizziness (Knight et al., 2014).

LATER IN PREGNANCY OR POST-DELIVERY

- Pre-eclampsia
- *Eclampsia*
- Haemolysis, elevated liver enzymes and low platelets (HELLP) syndrome is a haematological disturbance that can occur along with pre-eclampsia or as a discrete condition.

  Severe HELLP syndrome has significant maternal mortality and is an indication for referral for HDU care (Knight et al., 2016).

  As well as biochemical and haematological derangements, most women will present with right upper quadrant pain. HTN, proteinuria, nausea and vomiting are also common features.

  The only definitive treatment is delivery of the placenta with other management being purely supportive (Knight et al., 2016).
- Placental abruption
- Sepsis

HEADACHE

- Tension headache
  Usually bilateral
- Migraine
  Usually unilateral, may be preceded by aura (often visual), and can be associated with nausea, vomiting and photophobia
  May be new onset in pregnancy

- Drug-related

  Most commonly caused by vasodilators and in particular nifedipine used to treat pregnancy-induced hypertension (PIH)

Red flags suggesting more sinister underlying pathology include

- Sudden onset headache
- Associated neck stiffness
- Headache described by the woman as the worst headache she has ever had
- Any abnormal neurological signs (CMACE, 2011)

- Subarachnoid haemorrhage (SAH)

  Sudden, severe and often occipital. It is known as the 'thunderclap' headache.

  SAH can be the ultimate result of poorly controlled PIH.
- Cerebral venous thrombosis

  An unusually severe headache, which may be associated with focal signs (CMACE, 2011).

CARDIAC DISEASE

Cardiac disease has been the leading cause of maternal death since 2000. The increase in mortality due to cardiac disease has been attributed to increasing maternal age and increasing obesity (Knight et al., 2016).

The normal physiological changes that occur in pregnancy put women with pre-existing heart disease, especially those who are unable to increase their cardiac output, at risk of decompensation.

The majority of pregnant ladies who die due to heart disease are not identified as high risk and may not have a previous known diagnosis (Burt and Durbridge, 2009). In many obstetric patients who died, a diagnosis of heart disease was not considered (Knight et al., 2016).

The most common causes of cardiac mortality:

- Myocardial infarction – appropriate investigations and treatment should not be delayed because the lady is pregnant. The treatment of choice for acute coronary syndrome is primary percutaneous intervention (Steer et al., 2006).

- Peripartum cardiomyopathy – is a form of dilated cardiomyopathy usually diagnosed by echocardiogram. It is the presence of heart failure, with no other obvious cause, occurring from one month pre-delivery up to five months post-delivery (Knight et al., 2016).
- Aortic dissection – classically presents with severe tearing chest pain radiating to the back. The particular risk period is at full term and in the immediate post-partum period (Burt and Durbridge, 2009).

SEPSIS

Sepsis is a continuing area for improvement in clinical care and sepsis in the obstetric patient is no exception.

Pregnancy invokes an immune modulated state making obstetric patients susceptible to developing sepsis. Infections such as tuberculosis, pneumococcal meningitis pneumonia, and fungal infections can be amplified by the normal changes, which occur within the immune system during pregnancy. Pregnant or post-partum women are usually young and fit being able to withstand the physiological insults of sepsis appearing well until the point of collapse. This can occur with little warning and it is important to take seriously alterations in their vital signs, especially respiratory rate, as it may be an indication of the early stages of sepsis (Knight et al., 2014).

The definitions and tools for recognition of sepsis in general are covered in detail in a dedicated chapter. One difference in the obstetric patient population is the use of MEOWS (modified early obstetric warning score) not NEWS (national early warning score) to take account of the altered physiology of pregnancy. There is a range of clinical toolkits available on the UK Sepsis Trust website (http://sepsistrust.org/clinical-toolkit) specifically for women in pregnancy.

The causes of sepsis in the obstetric patient are slightly different to the general population and can be divided into 'obstetric' and 'non-obstetric'.

Obstetric		Non-obstetric
Gynaecological	Non-gynaecological	
Endometritis	Urinary tract infection	Pneumonia
Chorioamnionitis	Pyelonephritis	Influenza
Wound infection	Breast abscess/	Tuberculosis
• Caesarean section/ vaginal tear/episiotomy	mastitis	

Signs and symptoms of sepsis in the specific to the obstetric patient:

- Pyrexia > 38°C
- Sustained tachycardia > 100 bpm
- Breathlessness RR > 20
- Abdominal or chest pain
- Diarrhoea and/or vomiting
- Reduced or absent foetal movements, or absent foetal heart
- Spontaneous rupture of membranes or significant vaginal discharge
- Uterine or renal angle pain and tenderness
- Undue anxiousness, distressed or panic (Knight et al., 2011)

The treatment of sepsis in the obstetric patient is exactly as in the general population:

- Timely recognition
- Fast administration of antibiotics
- Senior review
- Adherence to the Sepsis Six protocol

EMBOLISM

THROMBOSIS AND THROMBOEMBOLISM

Thrombosis and thromboembolism remain the leading direct causes of maternal death (Knight et al., 2016).

Pregnancy is a hypercoagulable state increasing risk of thromboembolism. The risk period extends from the beginning of pregnancy to the end of the puerperium, including post miscarriage. Obesity in pregnancy amplifies the risk still further.

If a diagnosis of pulmonary embolism (PE) is considered, it should be investigated in the usual way with electrocardiography (ECG), chest X-ray, compression duplex ultrasonography, CT pulmonary angiography (CTPA) or VQ scan as clinically indicated. It is important to note that currently predictive tools for pulmonary embolism, such as the Wells score, are not validated for use in pregnancy and should not be used. The risk of CTPA and VQ scan is very small with VQ scanning potentially carrying a slightly increased risk of childhood cancer but lower risk of maternal breast cancer (Royal College of Obstetricians and Gynaecologists, 2013).

MANAGEMENT

Low molecular weight heparin is safe to use in pregnancy and should be dosed according to the lady's booking weight.

Thrombolysis should be considered.

AMNIOTIC FLUID EMBOLISM (AFE)

The presentation of AFE can be difficult to distinguish from other causes of maternal collapse, such as thromboembolism.

Effective resuscitation and high quality supportive care remains the essential common response despite the underlying cause.

	Amniotic fluid embolism	Pulmonary embolism
Timing of onset	During delivery	Any time
Early symptoms	Dyspnoea	Dyspnoea
	Anxiety	Cough
	Feeling cold	Haemoptysis
	Paraesthesia	Pleuritic pain
	Pain less likely	
Collapse	Highly likely	Less likely
DIC	Highly likely	Not present
ECG	Non-specific	Non-specific
Chest x-ray	Pulmonary oedema	Segmental collapse
	ARDS	Raised hemi-diaphragm
	Right atrial enlargement	Unilateral effusion
	Prominent pulmonary artery	
Arterial blood gases	Non-specific	Non-specific
CT pulmonary artery	Negative	Positive

Source: Adapted from a table produced by the Confidential Enquiry into Maternal and Child Health (CEMACH). *Saving Mothers' Lives: Reviewing Maternal Deaths to Make Motherhood Safer – 2003–2005.* The Seventh Report on Confidential Enquiries into Maternal Deaths in the United Kingdom. CEMACH, London, 2007.

PRE-ECLAMPSIA, ECLAMPSIA AND HELLP

PRE-ECLAMPSIA

It is defined as new onset hypertension presenting after 20 weeks of gestation with significant proteinuria. (Urine protein creatinine ratio [PCR] > 30 mg/mmol [or] a total protein excretion ≥ 300 mg per 24-hour collection of urine [or] two specimens of urine collected ≥ 4 hours apart with ≥2+ on the protein reagent strip.)

Signs and symptoms of severe pre-eclampsia:

- Headache
- Visual disturbances – blurring/flashing lights
- Upper abdominal pain – *epigastric pain presenting after 20 weeks should be treated as pre-eclampsia until proved otherwise*
- Nausea/vomiting
- Brisk deep tendon reflexes
- Sudden swelling of face, feet and hands
- Thrombocytopenia
- Coagulopathy
- Altered U&Es
- Increased serum urate
- Proteinuria
- Elevated urine PCR
- Low albumin
- Low glucose in severe cases

MANAGEMENT

A systolic BP >180 mmHg should be treated as a medical emergency (Knight et al., 2016). The ultimate sequelae of unmanaged HIP is intracranial haemorrhage.

Aggressively treat hypertension to keep BP < 150/100 by using one or more of the following, as the situation demands:

- Labetalol (PO or IV)
- Nifedipine (PO)
- Hydralazine (IV)
- Fluid restrict

Prevent seizures

- Magnesium

ECLAMPSIA

Eclampsia is convulsions associated with pre-eclampsia.
Magnesium is also used in the treatment of seizures.

HAEMORRHAGE

Haemorrhage is a common cause of maternal collapse.

It is important to remember that, in general, obstetric patients are young and healthy. Their large physiological reserve means that significant blood loss can occur before showing signs of decompensation.

CAUSES OF OBSTETRIC HAEMORRHAGE

Antepartum haemorrhage	Post-partum haemorrhage
Placental pathologies	Tone – uterine atony
Uterine rupture	Tissues – retained products
Ectopic pregnancy	Trauma – genital tract tears
	Thrombin – clotting abnormalities

MANAGEMENT

The general principles are the same as for any major haemorrhage – following the ABCDE approach.

There are, however, some specific treatment options in the management of uterine atony, which are listed as follows:

Pharmacological

- Oxytocin
- Ergometrine
- Carboprost
- Misoprostol

Surgical options

- B-Lynch (brace) suture
- Rusch balloon insertion
- Surgical ligation of the external iliac arteries
- Hysterectomy

IMPORTANT PHYSIOLOGICAL ALTERATIONS IN PREGNANT WOMEN

RESPIRATORY

- Capillary enlargement and mucosal congestion can occasionally narrow the airway causing dyspnoea.
- The diaphragm is elevated and the ribs 'splay' out making the mechanism of breathing predominantly diaphragmatic by term. Accessory respiratory muscles have limited impact in assisting when in respiratory distress.
- Functional residual capacity (FRC) is reduced by up to 20% and closing volume encroaches on FRC. This causes airway closure and hypoxia especially in the supine position. It is important to manage these patients in the 'ramped' position to assist oxygenation and ventilation.
- Oxygen consumption increases by up to 60% adding to the risk of hypoxia.
- Respiratory rate and minute ventilation increases making a $PaCO_2$ ~3.5 kPa and pH ~7.50 normal in pregnancy.
- Chest wall compliance reduces with lung compliance unchanged.

CARDIOVASCULAR

- Stroke volume and heart rate increase by up to 60% giving a cardiac output of ~8 L/min at term.
- Systemic vascular resistance decreases causing a reduction in DBP>SBP leading to a widened pulse pressure.
- Left ventricular mass increases, which may show as left axis deviation, ST depression and flat or inverted T waves on the ECG.
- Vena caval and aortic compression occurs from 20 weeks gestation. They cause a reduced venous return and increased afterload, resulting

in a decrease in cardiac output and a fall in BP. Utero-placental blood flow can also be compromised. If the woman needs to be in the supine position, it is vital that she is positioned with a minimum 15° left lateral tilt.

HAEMATOLOGY

- Normal Hb range for pregnancy 105 g/L at 28 weeks.
- Plasma volume increases by up to 50% at term.
- White blood cell (WBC) increases to $12 \times 10^9/L$ by term.
- Platelets reduce.
- Pregnancy is a hypercoagulable state making these women, especially with concurrent critical illness, at high risk of venous thromboembolism. Prophylactic anticoagulation is important and dosed according to the patient's weight.

RENAL

- Renal blood flow and glomerular filtration rate (GFR) increase by up to 50% reducing urea and creatinine levels.
- Glycosuria and proteinuria are common.

GASTROINTESTINAL

- Barrier pressure reduces due to raised intragastric pressure and increases the risk of aspiration. The risk of aspiration returns to normal 48 hours post-partum.
- Insulin levels increase but anti-insulin hormones like cortisol also increase, which can result in gestational diabetes (Wijayasiri et al., 2010).

CONCLUSION

Early recognition of severe illness in mothers remains challenging. The relative rarity of such events along with normal changes in physiology associated with pregnancy and childbirth exacerbates the problem. Timely involvement of senior clinical staff and effective multi-disciplinary team working are the key factors in providing high quality care to sick mothers. Relevant investigations or treatments for life-threatening conditions should not be delayed or postponed simply because the patient is pregnant or breastfeeding.

FURTHER READING

Burt, Christiana C., and Jacqueline Durbridge. "Management of Cardiac Disease in Pregnancy." *Continuing Education in Anaesthesia, Critical Care & Pain* 9, no. 2 (April 2009):44–47.

Centre for Maternal and Child Enquiries (CMACE). "Saving Mothers' Lives: Reviewing Maternal Deaths to Make Motherhood Safer: 2006–08." The Eighth Report on Confidential Enquiries into Maternal Deaths in the United Kingdom. *BJOG: An International Journal of Obstetrics & Gynecology* 118, Suppl. 1 (March 2011): 1–203.

Confidential Enquiry into Maternal and Child Health (CEMACH). *Saving Mothers' Lives: Reviewing Maternal Deaths to Make Motherhood Safer - 2003-2005*. The Seventh Report on Confidential Enquiries into Maternal Deaths in the United Kingdom. London: CEMACH; 2007.

Knight, Marian, Sara Kenyon, Peter Brocklehurst, Jim Neilson, Judy Shakespeare, and Jennifer J. Kurinczuk (eds.) on behalf of MBRRACE-UK. *Saving Lives, Improving Mothers' Care - Lessons Learned to Inform Future Maternity Care from the UK and Ireland Confidential Enquiries into Maternal Deaths and Morbidity 2009–12*. Oxford: National Perinatal Epidemiology Unit, University of Oxford, 2014.

Knight, Marian, Manisha Nair, Derek Tuffnell, Sara Kenyon, Judy Shakespeare, Peter Brocklehurst, and Jennifer J. Kurinczuk (eds.) on behalf of MBRRACE-UK. *Saving Lives, Improving Mothers' Care—Surveillance of Maternal Deaths in the UK 2012–14 and Lessons Learned to Inform Maternity Care from the UK and Ireland Confidential Enquiries into Maternal Deaths and Morbidity 2009–14*. Oxford: National Perinatal Epidemiology Unit, University of Oxford, 2016.

Knight, Marian, Derek Tuffnell, Sara Kenyon, Judy Shakespeare, Ron Gray, and Jennifer J. Kurinczuk (eds.) on behalf of MBRRACE-UK. *Saving Lives, Improving Mothers' Care - Surveillance of Maternal Deaths in the UK 2011–13 and Lessons Learned to Inform Maternity Care from the UK and Ireland Confidential Enquiries into Maternal Deaths and Morbidity 2009–13*. Oxford: National Perinatal Epidemiology Unit, University of Oxford, 2015.

Royal College of Obstetricians and Gynaecologists. "Ovarian Hyperstimulation Syndrome, Management (Green-top Guideline No. 5)." Royal College of Obstetricians and Gynaecologists, London, UK, February 2016.

Royal College of Obstetricians and Gynaecologists. "Thrombosis and Embolism during Pregnancy and the Puerperium, the Acute Management of (Green-top Guideline No. 37b)." Royal College of Obstetricians and Gynaecologists, London, UK, April 2015.

Steer, Philip J., Michael A. Gatzoulis, and Philip Baker (eds.). *Heart Disease and Pregnancy*. London: RCOG Press, 2006.

Wijayasiri, Lara, Kate McCombe, and Amish Patel. *The Primary FRCA Structured Oral Examination Study Guide 1*. Abingdon: Radcliffe Publishing, 2010.

50

The bariatric patient in intensive care

HELGA FICHTER

Steve, a 48-year-old patient of BMI 52 kg/m², was admitted to the intensive care unit (ICU) today. He is being treated for septic shock and acute kidney injury secondary to cellulitis of his legs. During your night shift, the nurse calls you to his bed. Steve is hypoxic; his breathing sounds noisy. He is slumped in his bed, sweating and restless. His arterial line is displaced. What would you do?

DEFINITION

Obesity is defined as a disease in which excess body fat has accumulated to such an extent that health may be adversely affected (WHO).

The extent of obesity is often described as body mass index (BMI) = weight (kg)/height² (m²). BMI $\geq$ 30 kg/m² defines obesity, BMI $\geq$ 40 kg/m² morbid obesity.

In addition to quantity, the distribution of fat is also important. The pattern can be predominantly gynaecoid located in the hip area or android located predominantly in the abdominal area. The latter poses a particular risk of adverse health consequences of obesity. Hence, obese patients are a heterogeneous group of individuals. You will see varying combinations of the findings discussed in this chapter.

Obesity is associated with physiological abnormalities, complications and comorbidities in several organ systems.

RESPIRATORY SYSTEM

UNFAVOURABLE RESPIRATORY MECHANICS IN THE FACE OF INCREASED OXYGEN CONSUMPTION

- Increased upper airway resistance
- Reduced chest wall compliance due to increased mechanical load from adipose tissue in the abdomen and chest wall

- Reduced lung compliance due to increased lung blood volume and small airway closure in the presence of reduced functional residual capacity
- Increased oxygen consumption owing to the metabolic requirement of excess adipose and supporting tissues as well as due to respiratory muscle oxygen demands resulting from increased work of breathing

These features mean that there is a mismatch between respiratory demand and capacity in comparison to the non-obese individual. In conditions of additional stress, this puts the obese patient at increased risk of hypoxia and respiratory pump failure.

OBSTRUCTIVE SLEEP APNOEA

It is characterised by frequent episodes of apnoea or hypopnoea, snoring and restlessness during sleep. Daytime symptoms caused by disrupted sleep are present as well. Complications include hypoxia, hypoxic pulmonary vaso-constriction leading to right ventricular failure and increased risk of isch-aemic heart disease.

Patients with obstructive sleep apnoea can be more sensitive to the effects of sedative drugs and opioids. Remember obese patients can have undiag-nosed obstructive sleep apnoea.

OBESITY HYPOVENTILATION SYNDROME

In severely obese patients, neural respiratory drive increases to compensate both for raised ventilatory load and inefficiency of the respiratory muscles. In obesity hypoventilation syndrome, this compensatory mechanism fails. Progressive desensitisation of the respiratory centre to carbon dioxide occurs resulting in hypoxia, hypercarbia and apnoeic events.

MANAGEMENT PRINCIPLES RELEVANT TO RESPIRATORY CARE

POSITIONING

The supine position is poorly tolerated. Obese patients should be sat up to 45°. This position presents the most favourable conditions with regards to work of breathing and oxygenation.

CPAP/NIV

Continuous positive airway pressure (CPAP) is a treatment in obstructive sleep apnoea. CPAP 10–15 cmH$_2$O is often required. Moreover, CPAP can increase lung and chest wall compliance and improve ventilation/perfusion matching. This results in lower work of breathing and improved oxygen saturation.

Similarly in non-invasive ventilation (NIV), higher levels of expiratory positive airway pressure (EPAP) and inspiratory positive airway pressure (IPAP) are commonly needed. Obese patients are at risk of sudden deterioration despite NIV. The initial management plan should make provision for this case.

INVASIVE MECHANICAL VENTILATION

The use of positive end-expiratory pressure (PEEP) has the same important role as end-expiratory pressure in NIV. Tidal volume should be based on the patient's ideal body weight rather than actual weight.

CARDIOVASCULAR SYSTEM

PHYSIOLOGY

Blood volume and extracellular fluid volume expand. Cardiac output increases to meet the requirement of raised baseline oxygen consumption. Left ventricular chamber size increases, left ventricular hypertrophy occurs in response to increased preload and hypertension. If the degree of hypertrophy does not keep pace with the degree of chamber dilatation, heart failure can ensue. Consider these points in fluid administration and haemodynamic management.

RISK OF CARDIOVASCULAR COMORBIDITY

Obesity is a risk factor for the metabolic syndrome: hypertension, insulin resistance, impaired glucose tolerance and dyslipidaemia. This predisposes to cardiovascular disease, non-fatty liver disease and diabetes mellitus.

RENAL SYSTEM

Obesity is established as a risk factor for chronic kidney disease. It has been identified as a risk factor for acute kidney injury in a number of critical care studies. Common equations for calculation of the glomerular filtration rate (GFR) may be inaccurate in obese patients.

NUTRITIONAL SUPPORT

Due to the catabolic state of critical illness, obese patients are at risk of protein–energy malnutrition, despite the presence of increased fat stores. Nutritional support can mitigate this and should be initiated as in all other patients. Nevertheless, established equations for energy requirements are not suitable for obese patients and the optimal way of estimating energy requirements is unclear.

IMMUNE SYSTEM CHANGES AND NOSOCOMIAL INFECTIONS

Pre-adipocytes and adipocytes produce molecules that stimulate macrophages and innate immune responses resulting in a chronic pro-inflammatory state. Obese patients could be at higher risk of nosocomial infections. Meticulous attention to infection prevention measures is important.

THROMBOEMBOLIC RISK

Thromboembolic risk is increased in obesity. Effective and safe prophylaxis is important. Higher than standard doses of low molecular weight heparins are required, but at present there is no universally accepted method of dose calculation due to limited scientific evidence. Some institutions have dosing guidelines in place.

PHARMACOLOGY/DRUG DOSING

It is challenging to account for obesity when dosing medications in the ICU. The physiological changes markedly affect distribution, protein binding and elimination of drugs. Data are often limited. For practical purposes, the following considerations might be helpful:

- Some drugs can be titrated to a rapidly observable effect, for example inotropes and vasopressors.

- Due to the possibility of drug accumulation in the excess tissue, elimination of sedative and opioid drugs administered by infusion can be prolonged. Therefore, in order to prevent prolonged sedation, it is important to strictly adhere to titration to the desired sedation score and interruption protocols.
- Some drugs can be titrated to their serum concentration levels or measured variables of effect (for example factor Xa).
- It is prudent to enlist help from other specialists as pharmacists, haematologists or microbiologists.

TECHNICAL AND ORGANISATIONAL ISSUES

BLOOD PRESSURE MONITORING

For non-invasive blood pressure monitoring, it is important to use the correct cuff size in order to avoid erroneously high readings due to too small cuff size. The length of the cuff bladder should be 80% and the width at least 40% of the circumference of the upper arm.

PLACEMENT OF VASCULAR ACCESS

Obtaining peripheral and central venous access can be difficult. Ultrasound can assist in these procedures.

AIRWAY MANAGEMENT

Apnoea is poorly tolerated because desaturation occurs more quickly in comparison to non-obese patients. This phenomenon, sometimes in combination with technical issues, can make airway management challenging.

Yet again positioning is important in this respect. The appropriate position for airway management will be ramping and if possible semi-sitting. Ramping describes the horizontal alignment of the tragus of the ear with the surface of the sternum. It is achieved by placing pillows and rolls under the head, neck and shoulders. In obese patients, meticulous attention to basic airway manoeuvres is crucial for maintenance of patency: chin lift, jaw thrust, using oral or nasopharyngeal airways. Mask ventilation can be more difficult. A two-provider technique may be useful.

In obese patients considered for invasive mechanical ventilation, it is essential that an airway management plan is always present. Likewise, extubation should be carefully planned for.

ORGANISATIONAL ISSUES

Bariatric patients often do not fit in standard-sized beds or chairs. It is important to know the weight limits of the equipment used in the unit, and have access to special bariatric beds, chairs, hoists, etc.

These patients are at increased risk of pressure sores and may need special pressure relieving mattresses designed for bariatric patients. Moving and handling (including transfers) may also be a challenge and require more trained staff, which may be difficult for smaller units. All units should have a plan for how to deal with the critically unwell bariatric patient.

HOW ABOUT STEVE?

You carry out a systematic assessment and find features of obstructive sleep apnoea. You also remember that body position is important so you arrange for him to have CPAP and to be sat up at 45°. You ensure that CPAP is set at a sufficiently high level. Steve starts to settle. Since his respiratory status is at risk of deterioration, you discuss his airway management plan with the team. Plus, you select a correctly sized cuff to measure his blood pressure pending reinsertion of his arterial line.

FURTHER READING

Shashaty, Michael G. S., and Renee D. Stapleton. "Physiological and Management Implications of Obesity in Critical Illness." *Annals of the American Thoracic Society* 11, no. 8 (October 2014): 1286–1297.

51

Post-ICU syndrome

JONATHAN PAIGE AND ANNA DENNIS

'Is he going to make a full recovery from this?'

Around 250,000 people are treated within UK intensive care units (ICUs) each year. As critical care standards improve, there are greater numbers of patients surviving critical illness. Our understanding of the psychological and physical morbidity after intensive care is increasing, and the concept of a post-ICU syndrome is developing.

WHAT IS POST-ICU SYNDROME?

Following treatment in the intensive care unit, patients can suffer with long-term physical, psychiatric and psychological problems, which can significantly impair survivors' quality of life. The post-ICU syndrome is complex as it can comprise any combination of these problems and can fluctuate over months and years following discharge from critical care.

Problems regularly reported include the following:

Physical	Non-Physical
Functional limitation	Cognitive dysfunction
General weakness	Post-traumatic stress
Fatigue	Depression
Weight loss	Anxiety
Hoarseness	Social isolation
Dyspnoea	Insomnia
Contractures	Loss of sexual relationships
Compression neuropathy	

PHYSICAL CONSEQUENCES

Survivors of critical illness regularly complain of a reduced functional status with impaired ability to perform simple activities of daily living, such as walking, dressing, bathing, making telephone calls and shopping. These effects are not only present on discharge but may also herald an acceleration in deterioration to perform these tasks over the following years. This increase in disability is seen across all populations no matter what the pre-morbid functional state and is associated with a loss of ability of patients to return to work and other normal activities.

NON-PHYSICAL CONSEQUENCES

Cognitive impairment following critical illness is thought to be due to direct hypoperfusion of the central nervous system leading to atrophy of the neural and myelin tissues. This is further exacerbated by inflammatory mediated degradation of these tissues and has been demonstrated with loss of grey-white differentiation within the brain of survivors of critical illness.

Cognitive impairment including immediate and delayed memory problems and ability to concentrate following ICU is extremely common with 40% of patients experiencing mild cognitive dysfunction at three months and persisting up to one year in 34%. New severe cognitive dysfunction equivalent to that of severe dementia is seen in up to 10% of patients treated for severe sepsis and can be persistent years after discharge from ICU. The effects seen affect all age groups; however, those with pre-existing cognitive impairment are worse affected.

Post-traumatic stress disorder (PTSD) is being increasingly recognised as a significant consequence of treatment in the critical care environment. Up to 40% of survivors complain of symptoms such as anxiety attacks, flashbacks, stress and insomnia for years after discharge from critical care. This is often associated with depression, decreased ability to work and difficulty forming social relationships.

The combination of the physical and nonphysical problems together leads to a significant effect on the patients' quality of life with many unable to return to normal function for a prolonged period of time or indeed ever. This has a cascade of consequences for the family and friends due to inability to work causing financial difficulty, change in personality putting strain on relationships, prolonged health problems, and in some cases, the need for family to act as informal carers changing family dynamics and putting even further strain on relationships and finances.

WHO IS LIKELY TO GET IT?

As post-ICU syndrome is such a broad-reaching and complex problem, it is difficult to define true risk factors. Certain factors predispose to some components of the syndrome whilst having no effect or even being protective against others; for example, increased age is related to worsening cognitive dysfunction and reduced functional capacity, but reduced incidence of PTSD.

Despite this, some factors are considered to be generally high risk including the following:

- Increased length of stay in ICU
- Increased time ventilated
- Increased time sedated
- Increased disease burden
- Increased number of organ failures
- Pre-existing disease
- Pre-existing cognitive dysfunction
- The use of benzodiazepines

WHAT CAN WE DO TO MANAGE IT?

Prevention of post-ICU syndrome necessitates a holistic approach to the patient's care involving multiple teams of healthcare professionals throughout the treatment process.

BEFORE ADMISSION TO ICU

Prevention begins before the patient even being admitted to the ICU where possible by explaining what the patient can expect in the ICU. This is relatively simple with elective post-surgery patients as visits to the unit can be arranged in advance. Unfortunately for many, admission to ICU is as an emergency so this is not possible. For this cohort, full explanation of why they are being admitted, what will be done to them and for them on the ICU is necessary if the patient has capacity and time allows. Where possible, family members or selected next of kin should be included in this as this allows them to reinforce what is being said.

DURING ICU STAY

Once a patient is admitted into the ICU, they should be assessed for their risks of developing physical and nonphysical problems as soon as feasibly possible as determined by their physiologic stability. Early rehabilitation during ICU stay can improve outcomes, reduce length of stay and help mitigate some of the features of post-ICU syndrome. Risks for developing problems are summarised below.

Risk of physical morbidity	Unable to mobilise out of bed
	Long ICU stay expected
	Neurological injury
	Cognitive dysfunction preventing independent exercise
	Oxygen requirement >35%
	Previous inability to mobilise short distances
Risk of non-physical morbidity	Nightmares
	Intrusive memories of traumatic events
	Anxiety and panic attacks
	Avoidance talking about illness

For those identified at risk, structured multidisciplinary plans should be made for rehabilitation. This should be decided in conjunction with members of the multi-disciplinary team (MDT), patients if possible, and their families. The rehabilitation plan should be holistic and address all areas of rehabilitation including medication review, nutritional support, physiotherapy, occupational therapy and psychology. As a team, long-term goals should be agreed with short-term goals being used as a bridge to achieving this.

Families should also be encouraged to keep a diary of the patient's stay in the ICU whether they are sedated or not as this can be referred to later to put context to anxieties and intrusive thought that the patient may have during their recovery and improve symptoms.

Regular sedation holds have also been shown to reduce the cognitive decline in patients on ICU. The mechanism is thought to be by improving communication with the patient, allowing them to recognise family members during visits and allowing some orientation between night and day.

FOLLOWING DISCHARGE FROM ICU

After discharge from the ICU, it is important that rehabilitation does not stop. Full detailed handover should take place between the ICU staff and the ward staff to ensure continuity of care. This should include explanation of treatment that the patient has received, what their current care needs are and a detailed description of rehabilitation status and goals of treatment.

Most ICUs now offer patients a clinic review, usually 1–3 months after their discharge from ICU. This is usually led by a senior nurse and allows further assessment of the patient's physical and non-physical symptoms following their ICU stay. The patient diary kept by the next of kin is regularly used as part of a 'debrief' to help discuss and explain intrusive thoughts, alleviate anxieties and explain misconceptions that the patient may have about their stay. Patients often report altered thoughts during their stay such as thinking ICU staff are trying to harm them or hearing discussions about other patients and thinking it relates to them. They may also have illusions, such as believing they are on a boat due to the rolling of the air mattress or believing they are falling when the bed is moved without prior explanation.

Further assessment regarding rehabilitation needs and referral for directed therapies, such as physiotherapy, cognitive behavioural therapy and psychology, as well as referral to medical specialities, such as ENT for assessment of persisting physical symptoms such as hoarseness and stridor, can also be made.

KEY LEARNING POINTS

- Patients admitted to ICU face a prolonged recovery with both physical and nonphysical consequences of their condition and the treatment, many have persistent or permanent cognitive decline following admission.
- Patients should be assessed for risk of developing long-term problems and rehabilitation started as soon as possible.
- Multidisciplinary team involvement is essential to rehabilitate and minimise morbidity after ICU admission.
- Care should be taken when in the vicinity of all ICU patients, sedated or not, as this is a major focus of disordered thoughts and anxiety in patients.

FURTHER READING

Angus, Derek C., and Jean Carlet, on behalf of the 2002 Brussels Roundtable participants. "Surviving Intensive Care: A Report from the 2002 Brussels Roundtable." *Intensive Care Medicine* 29, no. 3 (March 2003): 368–377.

Iwashyna, Theodore J., E. Wesley Ely, Dylan M. Smith, and Kenneth M. Langa. "Long-Term Cognitive Impairment and Functional Disability Among Survivors of Severe Sepsis." *Journal of the American Medical Association* 304, no. 20 (October 2010): 1787–1794.

National Institute for Health and Clinical Excellence (NICE). *Rehabilitation After Critical Illness.* Clinical Guideline CG83, National Institute for Health and Care Excellence, Manchester, UK, March 2009. www.nice .org.uk/guidance/cg83/evidence/full-guideline-242292349 (accessed 01 October 2016).

Pandharipande, Pratik P., Timothy D. Girard, James C. Jackson, Alessandro Morandi, Jennifer L. Thompson, Brenda T. Pun, Nathan E. Brummel, Christopher G. Hughes, Eduard E. Vasilevskis, Ayumi K. Shintani, Karel G. Moons, Sunil K. Geevarghese, Angelo Canonico, Ramona O. Hopkins, Gordon R. Bernard, Robert S. Dittus, and E. Wesley Ely, for the BRAIN-ICU Study Investigators. "Long-Term Cognitive Impairment after Critical Illness." *New England Journal of Medicine* 369, no. 14 (October 2013): 1306–1316.

52

End of life care in ICU

SARAH MILTON-WHITE AND LUCIE LINHARTOVA

'Mr Carter in Bed 10 was admitted with an infective exacerbation of interstitial lung disease. Despite completing a course of steroids and antibiotics, and trialling NIV, he has not improved and it has been decided to stop active treatment. This evening, he has become increasingly agitated and short of breath. What should I do?'

When patients are admitted to the intensive care unit (ICU) acutely unwell, it is for a period of stabilisation where the cause of deterioration is not always clear. Over time, it may become apparent that a patient has little chance of recovery either due to the acute pathology or co-existing health problems and decisions may be made to either limit or withdraw treatment.

In the United Kingdom, most people will die in the hospital and approximately 20% of patients admitted to ICU will die. Recognising a need to change from treatment with curative intent and moving towards managing symptoms is essential in ICU.

WHAT IS PALLIATIVE CARE?

Palliative care is defined by the World Health Organisation as 'an approach that improves the quality of life of patients and their families facing the problems associated with life-threatening illness, through the prevention and relief of suffering by means of an early identification and impeccable assessment and treatment of pain and other problems, physical, psychosocial and spiritual'. Palliative care can co-exist with treatment with curative intent.

IDENTIFYING PATIENTS

The decision to make the transition from treatment with curative intent to palliation requires careful planning and communication. There are many factors that need to be considered such as patient wishes, those of their surrogates when unable to communicate and the admitting parent team.

Good communication is essential to end of life care and needs to be centred on the patient and their contacts. There needs to be sufficient information about the rationale from switching the focus of care and what this will entail. This enables identification of key areas of concern and anxiety to be identified and alleviated. Involvement of palliative care services may not always be possible but will provide valuable support for the patient and those caring for them in addition to advice on symptom control and discharge planning.

Additional areas to consider:

- Stop unnecessary interventions
- Remove invasive lines that are not needed
- Spiritual and religious needs
- Visiting times

SYMPTOM CONTROL

PAIN

- Repositioning
- Identify reversible causes such as urinary retention
- Opioids
- Continue current regular analgesics and review doses

ANXIETY

- Reassurance
- Midazolam PRN

SECRETIONS

- Patient positioning and gentle suction
- Antimuscarinic such as hyoscine
- Monitor for drug side effects, such as urinary retention, dry mouth, agitation

NAUSEA AND VOMITING

- Consider potential causes: drug-induced, metabolic, intracranial, movement
- Unknown cause: administer haloperidol as first line, cyclizine as second line
- Regular and PRN doses

Dyspnoea

- Use of a fan
- Supplemental oxygen if hypoxic
- Opioids

END OF LIFE PRESCRIBING

- Stop all nonessential medication.
- Choose a suitable administration route.
- Consider infusions via subcutaneous or existing intravenous access based on existing doses, breakthrough requirements and to prevent withdrawal.

ANTICIPATORY PRESCRIBING

1. Analgesia
   a. Diamorphine 2.5–5 mg s/c hourly
   b. Morphine 2.5–5 mg
2. Anxiolytic
   a. Midazolam 2.5–5 mg s/c
   b. Levomepromazine 12.5–25 mg s/c
3. Secretions
   a. Hyoscine butylbromide 20 mg s/c (maximum 120 mg/24 hours)
   b. Glycopyrrolate 200 mcg s/c (maximum 1.2 mg/24 hours)
4. Breathlessness
   a. Morphine 2.5–5 mg s/c, IV
   b. May be more appropriate to commence infusion in some patients
5. Anti-emetic
   a. Haloperidol (drug-induced/biochemical)
   b. Metoclopramide (gastric stasis)
   c. Cyclizine (GI/CNS involvement)

The usage of anticipatory medication should be reviewed at least every 24 hours to ensure adequate symptom control.

PALLIATIVE CARE EMERGENCIES

HYPERCALCAEMIA

Hypercalcaemia can present with a variety of features ranging from confusion, nausea, thirst, and abdominal pain to seizures and coma. Treatment of hypercalcaemia will depend on prior history, patient preference and the appropriateness of treatment in advanced disease. Any calcium and vitamin D supplements should be stopped and IV rehydration commenced. Following adequate rehydration, bisphosphonates can be given such as pamidronate or zoledronic acid.

SVC OBSTRUCTION

SVC (superior vena cava) obstruction impedes venous return to the heart and can be caused by mediastinal lymphadenopathy, lung cancer and venous access. SVC obstruction can result in dyspnoea, facial swelling and plethora, headaches, dilated venous collaterals and positive Pemberton's sign. Initial treatment is aimed at reducing oedema, using dexamethasone followed by radiotherapy, chemotherapy or stenting.

MAJOR HAEMORRHAGE

Major haemorrhage can occur in some malignancies such as lung, head and neck and upper GI with the risk of bleeding affected by coagulopathy, proximity to major vessels, and infected or fungating lesions. The potential risk of major blood loss needs to be discussed carefully with the patient and carers to help reduce distress and formulate a management plan. In the event of a terminal bleed, the use of midazolam is recommended.

METASTATIC SPINAL CORD COMPRESSION

Spinal cord compression occurs in up to 10% of patients with cancer with most common primary sites being breast, prostate and lung. Suspicion should be raised in patients experiencing thoracic back pain, nocturnal pain and localised spinal tenderness, and neurological features such as limb weakness, sensory deficit and incontinence. Patients should be commenced on 16 mg dexamethasone orally, undergo MRI if suitable and be discussed with oncology for radiotherapy.

CASE REVIEW

- Review Mr Carter's notes and find out about events of admissions and discussions with patient and family/friends. Do the notes mention specific limitations?
- Review the patient: is there a reversible cause such as hypoxia or urinary retention?
- Review the drug chart: are any of the current medications a potential cause? Is Mr Carter on regular medications – such as opioids or benzodiazepines – that require dose titration?
- Start oxygen therapy if hypoxic and consider a fan to alleviate shortness of breath.
- Ensure anticipatory medication has been prescribed and administered such as morphine and midazolam.
- Communicate with family and friends present to explain what is happening and what your plan is.
- Talk to a senior: end of life care is not easy and it may help to share any concerns you may have.

KEY LEARNING POINTS

- Good communication is key.
- Stop all unnecessary interventions.
- Review medications regularly and prescribe anticipatory medications.
- Talk to someone if you have any doubts.

FURTHER READING

Cook, Deborah, and Graeme Rocker. "Dying with Dignity in the Intensive Care Unit." *New England Journal of Medicine* 370, no. 26 (June 2014): 2506–2514.

Gawande, Atul. *Being Mortal: Illness, Medicine and What Matters in the End.* New York, NY: Metropolitan Books, 2014.

National Institute for Health and Care Excellence (NICE). "Care of Dying Adults in the Last Days of Life." Clinical Guideline NG31, National Institute for Health and Care Excellence, December 2015. www.nice.org .uk/guidance/ng31 (accessed 24 October 2016).

West Midlands Palliative Care Physicians. "Guidelines for the Use of Drugs in Symptom Control: Palliative Care." www.wmpcg.co.uk (accessed 24 October 2016).

53

Brain stem death and organ donation

HUW TWAMLEY

'Doctor, I think the patient has just coned. Do you think they are suitable for organ donation?'

Although it is possible to donate some organs (kidney, liver) in life, organ donation in an intensive care setting usually occurs as cadaveric donation. Ethically, the donation process cannot cause/hasten the death of the patient (the 'dead donor rule'). Therefore, the patient has to be determined dead first before donation can proceed.

Death is defined as the irreversible loss of consciousness with the simultaneous loss of the ability to breathe. Tests to determine death vary between jurisdictions around the world. It can be determined either by neurological criteria or by circulatory criteria. The mode of determination also ultimately defines the organ donation process.

DONORS AFTER BRAIN STEM DEATH (DBD)

This follows a neurological definition of death. Brain stem death occurs through the disruption of blood supply either due to 'coning' or a direct cerebrovascular accident (clot/haemorrhage). It can also be caused by global hypoxia, such as occurs in a cardiac arrest.

WHAT IS CONING?

'Coning' is the process where the brain stem gets forced through the foramen magnum at the base of the skull due to increased intracranial pressure. This results in disruption of the blood supply to the brain stem and results in brain stem death. This disruption often manifests physiologically as marked hypertension and tachycardia followed by bradycardia and hypotension/ cardiovascular collapse. Pupils will be fixed and dilated. There will be no spontaneous breaths or cough reflex.

BRAIN STEM DEATH TESTING

To confirm death, two sets of tests have to be performed. The time of death is on completion of the first set of tests.

Each set is performed by two doctors; both need to be five years post-registration, and at least one doctor has to be a consultant.

The tests have three main stages, all of which have to be fulfilled.

PRE-CONDITIONS

- Apnoeic coma (no spontaneously triggered breaths on ventilator)
- Known cause of coma with brain damage consistent with diagnosis of brain stem death

- Known underlying cause
- Exclusions
- Reversible causes of coma excluded
- Exclude sedative drug effects (allowing for elimination half-life of drugs)
- No neuromuscular blockade
- Temp > 34°C
- Mean arterial blood pressure > 60 mmHg (this may require CVS support including fluids and inotropes due to loss of sympathetic activity in brain stem dead patients)
- PaO_2 > 10 kPa
- $PaCO_2$ < 6.0 kPa
- pH 7.35–7.45
- Electrolytes sodium 115–160 mmol/L
  - Potassium > 2.0 mmol/L
  - Magnesium 0.5–3.0 mmol/L
  - Phosphate 0.5–3.0 mmol/L
- Normal endocrine levels (assays only if clinical suspicion)

CLINICAL EXAMINATION

Examination looks at the cranial nerve and respiratory centre function of the brain stem.

- Pupils are fixed and do not respond to light.
- Absent corneal reflexes (cotton wool/gauze dragged across cornea with no facial reaction).
- Absent oculovestibular reflexes (instilling at least 50 mL ice-cold water into each ear).
- No motor response within cranial nerve distribution to painful stimulus (usually supra-orbital pressure).
- Note peripheral movements may result from spinal reflexes. These do not invalidate the tests.
- Absent gag reflex (usually spatula introduced into posterior pharynx).
- Absent gag reflex (usually suction catheter inserted into ET tube to carina).

APNOEA TEST

The respiratory centre in the brain stem is stimulated by a respiratory acidosis not by hypoxia. For the tests to be valid, oxygenation needs to be maintained and the tests should only start with a CO_2 >6.0 and a pH <7.4 (may need a higher CO_2 to produce acidosis in chronic respiratory patients).

- Ventilated patients will be pre-oxygenated for at least five minutes and then hypoventilated (decreased tidal volume and/or respiratory rate) to allow the CO_2 and pH to be in the correct range.
- The patient is then disconnected from the ventilator whilst being oxygenated with either oxygen via a suction catheter connected to oxygen supply or via Water's circuit.
- *If* the patient becomes hypoxic or cardiovascular unstable, then the test has to be terminated.
- No respiratory activity should be observed for five minutes and the $PaCO_2$ should rise by more than 0.5 kPa.
- The ventilator is then reconnected.
- Two full sets of tests are required with no specified time interval between them.

If suitable for organ donation and there is family consent, then the patient goes to theatre for retrieval on the ventilator and with the circulation still intact.

Donation of kidneys, liver, small bowel, pancreas and, importantly, cardio-respiratory organs can be donated.

DONATION AFTER CIRCULATORY DEATH (DCD)

This is considered in patients in whom treatment is being withdrawn and who do not fit the criteria for brain stem testing. Practically, these are often ventilated patients with neurological injuries, such as subarachnoid haemorrhage (SAH), or head injuries but occasionally some non-invasively ventilated patients are suitable.

As these patients are alive, organ donation can only occur if they die once treatment is withdrawn and importantly if the dying process is not prolonged.

Warm ischaemic injury occurs to the organs that will be potentially donated and usually the patient needs to die *within three hours of withdrawal* for the organs to be suitable to be transplanted.

This means that a significant number of patients do not go on to donate because they do not die in time.

The process is as follows in a suitable patient with family consent for organ donation.

- Treatment withdrawn (in intensive care or theatre complex/anaesthetic room depending on local hospital policy).
- Patient dies (within suitable time).
- Death confirmed by circulatory criteria.
- Patient moved quickly into operating room where retrieval team waiting.
- Laparotomy (within ten minutes of loss of circulation).
- Inferior vena cava (IVC) and aorta cannulated, and cold cardioplegia-type solution infused to stop metabolic activity of organs to prevent further ischaemic damage.
- Organs retrieved.

Organs donated can include kidneys, liver, pancreas, and in recent developments, cardiorespiratory organs.

As can be seen from the time-critical process above, it is very important that death is confirmed in a timely but appropriate and thorough manner.

Assessment for organ donation suitability

- Organ donation suitability can be determined only by the Specialist Nurse for Organ Donation (SNOD).
- All hospitals should have a policy for referral for the SNODs, which should be available on your unit.
- Guidance from the National Institute for Health and Care Excellence (NICE) regarding organ donation recommends that all patients who fit the following criteria should be referred for assessment of suitability of organ donation.
- There is an intention to withdraw life-limiting treatment.
    - Or an intention to test for brain stem death.
- It is important to know whether a patient is suitable for organ donation as this will affect the timing and, in some cases, the place of withdrawal.
- It is therefore good practice to refer before discussions with the family.
- The Organ Donor Register (ODR) should be checked (often this is done by the SNOD) as this is an expression of the patient's previously held wishes.
- In Wales, where 'presumed consent' has been in place since December 2015, patients may have 'opted out' of donation.
- Families/next of kin need to give their consent for organ donation to occur.

- Consent rate is higher when the ODR status is known but occasionally families will override the patient's wishes.
- It is important that families are approached in collaboration with the SNOD, in a sensitive manner at a time when they have understood and accepted either treatment withdrawal or the implication of brain stem death tests.
- It is often the case that there is a short hiatus between the discussions above and then approaching the families about donation, so that they have time to process the potential loss of their loved one.
- Consent rate is significantly higher when the SNOD is involved in the approach as they are trained in approaching families better skilled at addressing families concerns and talking about the positives of organ donation.

CLINICAL PRIORITIES

- Due to the significant physiological effects of brain stem death, patients will often need optimising so that they are suitable and stable for testing.
- Review intravascular fluid status and correct hypovolaemia.
- Start inotropes/vasopressors if necessary for a MAP target 60–80 mmHg.
- Use cardiac output monitoring if still unstable.
- Look for diabetes insipidus.
- If urine output > 4 mL/kg/hr, give 0.5–1 mcg bolus of desmopressin.
- Replace/correct electrolytes, especially sodium.
- Ensure lung-protective ventilation.
- Maintain normothermia.

Approaching families about donation should only be done by doctors or specialist nurses trained in approaching families.

DONOR OPTIMISATION

Once consent has been obtained from the family and brain stem death has been confirmed, the emphasis changes to optimising the condition of the potential organ transplants.

In addition to the points above, also consider:

- Methylprednisolone (dose 15 mg/kg; max 1 g)
- Vasopressin (0.5–4 units/hour) (can be used prior to testing)
- Liothyronine infusion at 3 units per hour if unstable
- Insulin infusion to keep blood sugar 4–10 mmol/L

HOW DO YOU RESPOND TO THE NURSE'S QUESTION?

- Refer to the SNOD, in line with your local unit policy.
- Optimise the patient for brain stem testing including stopping sedation.
- Focus on intravascular assessment and electrolyte correction.
- Look for and treat any diabetes insipidus.
- Document actions clearly including intention to brain stem test.

KEY LEARNING POINTS

- There are two forms of cadaveric donation dependent on the mode of death.
- Do not approach families about organ donation but make sure they are referred to the SNODs.
- Patients need optimising for brain stem tests to be performed.
- Donor optimisation can result in more patients benefitting from transplanted organs.

FURTHER READING

Organ Donation and Transplantation (National Health Service). "Donation after Brainstem Death (DBD): Donor Optimisation Extended Care Bundle." Document. http://odt.nhs.uk/pdf/dbd_care_bundle.pdf.

Simpson, Peter, David Bates, Stephen Bonner, Kate Costeloe, Len Doyal, Sue Falvey, Jean Gaffin, Robin Howard, Nick Kane, Colin R. Kennedy, Ian Kennedy, Steven Kerr, Alex Manara, John Pickard, Keith Rolles, and Alasdair Short. "A Code of Practice for the Diagnosis and Confirmation of Death." Report for the Academy of Medical Royal Colleges. London, UK, 2008.

Index